CHILD PSYCHIATRY
Treatment and Research

Child Psychiatry
Treatment and Research

Edited by

MAE F. McMILLAN, M.D.

Early Childhood Therapy Clinic,
Texas Research Institute of Mental Sciences

and

SERGIO HENAO, M.D.

Chief, Family Psychiatry Section,
Texas Research Institute of Mental Sciences

PROCEEDINGS OF THE TENTH ANNUAL SYMPOSIUM,
SEPTEMBER 29 - OCTOBER 1, 1976

TEXAS RESEARCH INSTITUTE OF MENTAL SCIENCES
HOUSTON, TEXAS

BRUNNER/MAZEL, *Publishers* • New York

Library of Congress Cataloging in Publication Data

Main entry under title:
Child psychiatry.

  Includes bibliographies and index.
  1. Child psychotherapy—Congresses.   I. McMillan, Mae F., 1936-   II. Henao,
Sergio, 1940-   III. Texas Research Institute of Mental Sciences.
RJ504.C47   618.9'28'914   77-2228
ISBN 0-87630-149-9

Published by
BRUNNER/MAZEL, INC.
19 Union Square West, New York, N. Y. 10003

Contributors

MICHAEL BAIZERMAN, Ph.D.

Associate Professor, Center for Youth Development and Research, and Associate Professor, Maternal and Child Health, School of Public Health, University of Minnesota, St. Paul, Minnesota

LESTER BAKER, M.D.

Director, Clinical Research Center, Children's Hospital of Philadelphia; Professor of Pediatrics, University of Pennsylvania, School of Medicine, Philadelphia, Pennsylvania

T. BERRY BRAZELTON, M.D.

Director, Child Development Unit, Children's Hospital Medical Center, Boston, Massachusetts

VICTOR G. CICIRELLI, Ph.D.

Professor of Developmental Psychology, Department of Psychological Sciences, Purdue University, West Lafayette, Indiana

DAVID B. EAGLE, M.D.

Fellow, Child Development Unit, Children's Hospital Medical Center, Boston, Massachusetts

NORMAN GARMEZY, Ph.D.

Professor of Psychology, University of Minnesota, Minneapolis,

Minnesota; Clinical Professor of Psychiatry (Psychology), School of Medicine, University of Rochester, Rochester, New York

RICHARD GREEN, M.D.

Professor, Departments of Psychiatry and Psychology, State University of New York at Stony Brook, Stony Brook, New York

HENRY GRUNEBAUM, M.D.

Director, Family and Group Psychotherapy Training, The Cambridge Hospital, Cambridge, Massachusetts; Associate Clinical Professor of Psychiatry, Harvard Medical School; Director, Family Planning and Counseling Services, Massachusetts Mental Health Center, Boston, Massachusetts

SAUL I. HARRISON, M.D.

Professor of Psychiatry, The University of Michigan Medical Center, Children's Psychiatric Hospital, Ann Arbor, Michigan

SERGIO HENAO, M.D.

Chief, Family Psychiatry Section, Texas Research Institute of Mental Sciences, Houston, Texas

MARGARET MORGAN LAWRENCE, M.D.

Supervising Psychiatrist, Developmental Psychiatry Service, Division of Child Psychiatry, Department of Psychiatry, Harlem Hospital Center; Associate Clinical Professor of Psychiatry, College of Physicians and Surgeons, Columbia University, New York, New York

RONALD LIEBMAN, M.D.

Psychiatrist-in-Chief, Children's Hospital of Philadelphia; Acting Medical Director, Philadelphia Child Guidance Clinic; Assistant Professor of Child Psychiatry and Pediatrics, University of Pennsylvania, School of Medicine, Philadelphia, Pennsylvania

GERALD E. McCLEARN, Ph.D.

Professor of Psychology and Director, Institute for Behavioral Genetics, University of Colorado, Boulder, Colorado

MAE F. McMILLAN, M.D.

Early Childhood Therapy Clinic, Texas Research Institute of Mental Sciences; Clinical Associate Professor of Psychiatry, Department of Psychiatry, University of Texas Medical School at Houston; Associate Professor of Psychiatry, Baylor College of Medicine, Houston, Texas

SALVADOR MINUCHIN, M.D.

Director, Family Therapy Training Center, Philadelphia Child Guidance Clinic; Professor of Child Psychiatry and Pediatrics, University of Pennsylvania, School of Medicine, Philadelphia, Pennsylvania

SALLY PROVENCE, M.D.

Professor of Pediatrics and Child Psychiatry and Director, Yale University Child Study Center, Yale University, New Haven, Connecticut

LEE N. ROBINS, Ph.D.

Professor of Psychology, Department of Psychiatry, Washington University School of Medicine, St. Louis, Missouri

BERNICE ROSMAN, Ph.D.

Philadelphia, Pennsylvania
Director of Research, Philadelphia Child Guidance Clinic,

MILTON F. SHORE, Ph.D.

Associate Chief, Mental Health Study Center, National Institute of Mental Health, Adelphi, Maryland; Adjunct Professor, Catholic University of America, Washington, D.C.

ROBERT L. SPRAGUE, Ph.D.

Director, Institute for Child Behavior and Development, and Professor, School of Basic Medical Sciences, Department of Psychology and Department of Special Medical Education, University of Illinois, Champaign, Illinois

JUDITH S. WALLERSTEIN, M.S.W.

Lecturer, School of Social Welfare, University of California, Berkeley, California

ERIC WISH, Ph.D.

Postdoctoral Fellow, Department of Psychiatry, Washington University School of Medicine, St. Louis, Missouri

PETER H. WOLFF, M.D.

Professor of Psychiatry, Harvard Medical School, and Director of Psychiatric Research, The Children's Hospital Medical Center, Boston, Massachusetts

Contents

ix

PART III
THERAPEUTIC INTERVENTION RESEARCH

PART IV
RESEARCH ON THE FAMILY

PART V
SOCIALIZATION RESEARCH

Introduction

Childhood is a unique, dynamic stage in a person's growth, not merely an anteroom to maturity. The child is a person in his or her own right, the subject of investigation by many disciplines—cultural anthropology, psychology, sociology, psychoanalysis, pediatrics, and pedagogy.

A closer scrutiny of children's needs from a normal developmental view has broadened and made more meaningful the concept of mental health as applied to children. The estimate that from ten to fourteen percent of all children in the United States are in need of some type of mental health service shows that primary prevention must be given a major part of our attention and efforts.

There are identifiable individuals who have heightened potential for later disorder. In this volume research in such fields as genetics, neurophysiology, neuropsychology, and comparative child development is singled out for special emphasis to clarify the many correlations between risk and vulnerability.

Both basic research and applied research in the biological, behavioral, and social sciences have produced pertinent data for treatment as well as for primary prevention. If we are to continue to grapple effectively with the vagaries of child development and child psychopathology, a national research climate that encourages the productivity and expands the opportunities of the individual investigator must be maintained. The interdisciplinary team approach to research problems over time seems to yield the most useful data. Such research projects, undertaken with sufficiently large samples of children from various kinds of background, do seem feasible and necessary, especially for this age group.

The tenth annual symposium of the Texas Research Institute of Mental Sciences was the first one in the history of these symposia to discuss treatment and research in child psychiatry. It reflected a new emphasis in research and an expansion of children's services at the institute. It is a pleasure for us to introduce the volume resulting from this symposium because it contains an outstanding collection of papers dealing with a variety of concerns in the field.

The chapters are clustered around main subjects. In *Biological Foundations of Child Development,* Peter Wolff and Gerald Mc-Clearn discuss the importance of maturational and genetic factors in the study and evaluation of children. Wolff points out that, "Since child psychiatrists neither can, nor should, interfere with maturational rate, their essential contribution to primary prevention . . . may be to protect children against society's biologically unsound demands that children should conform to the bell-shaped curve, and to inform parents, teachers, and colleagues about the inherent strength conferred on any society when it encourages individual variations."

The section on *Risk Research and Primary Prevention* includes a chapter by David Eagle and T. Berry Brazelton on the assessment of infants at risk, using the now well-known Brazelton scale. The authors believe that it is not only the child who may be at risk, but the environment as well, and they suggest the development of evaluations of infant-mother interactions, since the behavior of the child is only one aspect of a complex, mutually influencing interplay between infant and caretaker.

Norman Garmezy continues the discussion, pointing out the tremendous methodological and human problems involved in risk research, especially of schizophrenia. He points to Manfred Bleuler's studies of the children of schizophrenic parents, which show how remarkably adaptive and competent many of these children turned out to be. Garmezy pleads for a shift from the study of the "vulnerable" and disturbed child to the study of the "invulnerable" and adaptive one.

In a parallel view, Margaret Morgan Lawrence emphasizes the positive and often unnoticed familial and cultural values of children raised in the risky environment of the inner city. "The history, culture, and myths of a people, 'the stuff of life itself,' can make available to those who share it, their own ego strengths . . . ," she writes.

In *Therapeutic Intervention Research,* Saul Harrison gives a scholarly review of eclecticism in child therapy and shows how many advances in treatment of psychiatric disturbances originated in child psychiatry. And as he points out, "the choice of treatment stems far more often from the therapeutic-professional system's institutional or personal preferences than from an assessment of the recipients' individual differences."

Milton Shore presents his fascinating results of ten years of psychotherapeutic intervention with adolescent delinquents. He discusses the pitfalls of traditional psychotherapy with this difficult population and describes how he and his associates arrived at what he considers a successful approach. On the scientific evaluation of psychotherapy he makes an eloquent comment: "While the search for a simple intervention technique has been fruitless, there has also been a vain search to find an easy test for the profound changes that result from psychotherapeutic intervention . . . it seems that we have confused clarity of thinking with narrowness of vision and have often resorted to what is measurable, rather than what is meaningful."

The section is completed by an extensive review of psychopharmacotherapy for children by Robert Sprague who analyzes the complex issues of prescribing medication for minimally brain-disordered and mentally retarded children.

Research on the Family includes a report by Ronald Liebman, Salvador Minuchin and associates at the Philadelphia Child Guidance Clinic on the group's innovative work in what has become known as structural family therapy. Henry Grunebaum makes two interesting suggestions: (1) to designate a "family mental health doctor" who would act as an ombudsman for families in the mental health system and (2) to offer family planning and contraceptive services to clients of mental health agencies. Victor Cicirelli reviews the subject of sibling effects on cognitive styles as part of the socialization process and finds interesting differences according to the sex of the child.

In *Socialization Research,* Sally Provence, who is well-known for her work with children in institutions, reviews the psychoanalytic and developmental literature on mother-infant interaction and points out the importance of this relationship as a system in which both child and parent undergo their own developmental processes.

Lee Robins presents a fascinating longitudinal study of childhood deviance in 223 urban black men from birth to 18, exploring possible developmental patterns of deviant behavior. Richard Green, in the chapter on atypical sex-role development in children, outlines some surprising and controversial issues: for example, what are the effects of homosexual parents' keeping and raising their children?

In the final section, *Special Research Problems,* Judith Wallerstein reports her findings of another longitudinal work, "Responses of the Preschool Child to Divorce: Those Who Cope." Like Garmezy, she shows us that studying invulnerable children, or those who cope, is at least as important as research with those who do not. Her observations lead her to say, "there is little evidence in our study that preschool children who are able to articulate their feelings necessarily do better than those who deny, avoid, or otherwise shy away from such expression." If confirmed, these findings would obviously have tremendous influence on crisis and intervention theories.

The last chapter is by Michael Baizerman, who analyzes the difficulties of building a bridge between researchers and practitioners, illustrating the point with the problem of helping pregnant adolescents. Again, he suggests that more might be learned from the study of successes instead of failures; in this case, why do some adolescents become pregnant while others do not?

Thus, one of the messages of these writers is the need to study more of the children who cope, the competent children. Or, to paraphrase Jacques May's metaphor of the three dolls, Why does the glass doll break, the plastic one bear a permanent scar, and the steel doll ring with a pleasant sound—even though all have been struck with a hammer equally hard? Obviously we have only begun to look at this question, since most of our past investigations have been of pathology. We hope that books like this one will enrich understanding of ways in which children can be helped to cope.

ACKNOWLEDGMENTS

For their financial support of the symposium we are grateful to the George and Mary Josephine Hamman Foundation, Hogg Foundation for Mental Health, Merck Sharpe & Dohme Postgraduate Program, New England Nuclear Corporation, Alvin and Lucy Owsley Foundation, Sandoz Pharmaceuticals, and Tenneco Inc. Thanks to Joseph Schoolar, director of the Texas Research Institute, for his guidance of the symposium series, and to Frank Womack and the institute staff for arrangements and organization.

Thanks to Julie Smoorenburg, Margaret Dawkins, Lillie Oliver, and many others who did the tremendous secretarial and clerical work and who, with some volunteers, helped us staff the symposium.

Special thanks to Lore Feldman for her assistance in planning the symposium and for editing the manuscript with Marsha Recknagel's help.

Leading the discussions and animating them with their own brief reports, questions and clarifications were Roy N. Aruffo, William Harrison Boylston, Hilde Bruch, C. Glenn Cambor, Murdina M. Desmond, Douglas B. Hansen, James C. Heald, Lawrence G. Hornsby, Irvin A. Kraft, Richard B. Pesikoff, Carl M. Pfeifer, Manuel C. Ramirez, James S. Robinson, Charles I. Scott, Jr., Alberto C. Serrano, and George Wawrykow. Many thanks to them all.

MAE F. MCMILLAN
SERGIO HENAO

CHILD PSYCHIATRY
Treatment and Research

Part I

BIOLOGICAL FOUNDATIONS OF CHILD DEVELOPMENT

1

Maturational Factors in Behavioral Development

PETER H. WOLFF, M.D.

While considering the many ways in which developmental research might contribute to the practice of preventive child psychiatry, I thought it advisable to consult physicians with a primary responsibility for the mental health of children, who could define for me the most pressing health problems in the field.

Although there was unanimous disagreement about the clinical priorities, all agreed that the demands for child psychiatric services cover such a broad spectrum of disciplines that the field is defined more by what child psychiatrists do than by what they are trained to do. They also agreed that prevention is probably the only long-range solution, and that in order to respond appropriately to current needs, child psychiatrists must shift their primary focus from the suburban play-therapy office to hospital wards, pediatric outpatient departments, schools, custodial institutions, and the community at large.

What constitutes effective prevention in child psychiatry, however, remained obscure, since adequate preparation for the task would require, in addition to conventional clinical training, some knowledge of population and cytogenetics, biochemistry, pharmacology, and toxicology; neuropathology, neurology, and neuroendocrinol-

Work for this report was completed with support from USPHS Research Grants MH 18332-04 and HD 02-0773, and Career Scientist Award MKH 3461.

3

ogy; development, education, and neuropsychology; special education, sociology, and forensic psychiatry; and for those committed to
long-term solutions, it would require disciplined training in community work and political action.

Considering the scope of problems that confront the field, this
chapter cannot hope to be exhaustive. I will therefore confine my
discussion to some recent advances in developmental research that
are substantially modifying current theoretical formulations about
the ontogenesis of behavior.

Two basic premises will serve as my point of departure:

1. The developing organism is not a miniature version of the
mature form. Its rules of behavioral organization and transformation differ qualitatively from those relevant for the adult.

2. The proper frame of reference for systematic studies in clinical
child psychiatry is defined by the biological and psychobiological
disciplines, particularly developmental biology. This premise might
be challenged by those who maintain that the proper concern of
child psychiatry is the symbolization of experience and the social-
affective development of children, whereas a zealous preoccupation
with mechanistic explanations of behavior threatens to reduce the
core of human experience to meaningless fragments. Although this
view has much to recommend it in this age of relentless empiricism
and mechanistic psychology, it will by itself not resolve the crucial
issues of prevention which are the focus of this volume.

In keeping with the two premises, I will therefore focus on some
recent advances in the biology of behavioral development.

Comprehensive accounts of development agree in principle that
biology and experience are always reciprocally determined vectors,
and that their interaction can never be entirely isolated in clinical
assessments or experimental design. In the conduct of concrete experiments, developmental psychology is therefore inclined to apply a
strategy of "holding one vector constant" while investigating the
effects of the other—a strategy which is productive when it alter-
nates between observations of biological phenomena and of the in-

fluences of psychological experience to explain behavioral development. In practice, however, empirical research in developmental psychology has generally neglected the biological vector, concentrating almost exclusively on experience as the sufficient cause to explain developmental variations.

Where developmental psychology recognizes biological maturation as an important variable, it has usually applied chronological age as the independent variable, thus making the tacit assumption that maturation is as uniform in its relation to physical time as chronological age. Yet, Wohlwill (1973) has argued persuasively that chronological age is an artificial measure based on physical rather than biological time. He suggests that the circular conclusions which result from use of chronological age as the independent variable of development can be circumvented if we substitute physical or physiological growth measures.

Tanner's studies of physical development (1970) demonstrate how greatly children of the same chronological age may vary in maturational state; like Wohlwill, he recommends physiological indices of maturity or "developmental age" as the preferred independent variables. Very few biological measures of maturation, however, have been shown to relate specifically to the development of behavior. Skeletal growth curves are a useful first approximation, but their relation to brain maturation is indirect and their relevance to psychological development has been demonstrated only in correlations. Direct measures of human brain growth are not sufficiently precise at present to reveal how the maturation of brain functions determines specific aspects of behavioral development (Purpura, 1973). Despite an enduring debate about the relation between myelinogenesis and brain function (McKhann, Coyle, and Benjamins, 1973), central nervous system myelinogenesis probably provides the best overall map of regional variations in human brain maturation that is currently available. The meticulous morphological studies by Yakovlev and Lecours (1967) and Rakic and Yakovlev (1968), for example, indicate that major inter- and intrahemispheric association pathways do not complete their growth until some time between 4 and 12 years of age. Assuming that myelination is an indirect clue to the onset of function, it should follow that maturation influences behavioral development throughout infancy and childhood, particularly as development is influenced by the progressive lateralization of cerebral functions and by increased inter- and intrahemispheric coordinations (Trevarthen, 1974).

From a clinical perspective, severe malnutrition during gestation and early infancy demonstrates the complexity of relations between maturation and behavioral development. Significant correlations between infantile malnutrition and intellectual deficits in later childhood have been reported by numerous investigators (Cravioto, DeLicardie, and Birch, 1966; Ricciuti, 1973). Others have concluded that, except in the severest cases, there are no irreversible effects. They tend to attribute the positive correlations to confounding factors of social class, sensory deprivation, somatic illness, and family disorganization which so often accompany malnutrition, especially in populations of the developing countries where such malnutrition studies are usually conducted (Ricciuti, 1973).

However, the presence or absence of late psychological effects of early malnutrition cannot be decided on the basis of currently available evidence. The outcome measures in nearly all human malnutrition studies have been standardized psychometric tests, which are probably too crude to detect any but extreme growth-retarding effects. Experimental animal studies indicate, for example, that regions of the central nervous system growing at a fast rate are more vulnerable to exogenous growth-retarding factors than regions which have already passed the maximal growth spurt or have not yet started it (Dobbing, 1968; Dobbing and Sands, 1971). The profile of behavioral impairments as a result of pre- or postnatal malnutrition would therefore depend on the timing of malnutrition in ontogenesis as well as on its severity. In addition to the delayed onset of a psychological function represented by one specific vulnerable region of the developing brain, regional delay in one sector may modify the epigenetic organization among adjacent structures, and result in a behavioral outcome that is manifested as a qualitative variation in the profile of performance characteristics. Experimental evidence on mammalian as well as nonmammalian species indicates, for example, that surgical or chemical ablation of lateral brain structures during fetal life may be compensated by the growth of new branching fiber tracts from homologous contralateral groups of cell bodies, as if to maintain or restore structural integrity. Since many of the new fiber tracts are functionally competent, one might predict profound and irreversible effects not only on brain architecture, but also on the overall organization of behavior, although such effects have not been studied in great detail. Assuming that malnutrition before or shortly after birth has selective regional effects, the developmental organization of behavior patterns should be modified in ways that are not detectable by the conventional psychometric assessment or discrete psychological "tests"—except in the extreme case, which provides no useful information about the details of brain-behavior relations (Wolff, 1970b).

Early malnutrition is only one among many implicated or suspected biological factors that interfere selectively with regional brain maturation. We know relatively little about the behavioral outcome of pre- or postnatal exposure to heavy metals or other toxic substances with mutagenic effects, or about the "subclinical" effects of viral infections and pharmacologic agents on brain development during fetal life. Each growth-retarding agent will have its main effects at a different stage in ontogenesis, and the behavioral outcome will vary qualitatively with the nature of the exogenous agent as well as the biological time of exposure. There is, for example, some evidence that prenatal rubella infections may either mimic such clinical syndromes as infantile autism, for which a psychogenic etiology is assumed, or be a direct causal factor (Chess, 1971; Ornitz and Ritvo, 1976). To what extent exogenous factors interfering with maturation may contribute to other psychiatric syndromes is a matter that I believe deserves our most careful attention.

The study of behavioral outcome after pathological growth retardation demonstrates the interactions between maturation and mental development most dramatically. By itself, however, such evidence does not constitute a secure base from which to draw conclusions about maturational factors in normal mental development. Clinical psychiatry provides many examples in which extrapolations from the pathological to the normal case have led us to draw erroneous conclusions. In the case of maturational variations, such extrapolations may cause us to label as deviant or pathological those normal biological variations that conflict with arbitrary social expectations, and motivate us to impose elaborate enrichment procedures in order to homogenize children according to some arbitrary social criterion (Wolff, 1970a). We must, therefore, also find models that demonstrate the effects of maturation on normal behavioral development.

The analysis of behavioral sex differences can, I believe, provide such a model. On the average, girls are physically more mature than boys throughout the period of childhood and adolescence. Although the differences are most evident during periods of rapid growth like the prepubertal growth spurt (Tanner, 1970) or the "5-7 shift" (White, 1970), similar sex differences in physical maturity are already evident at birth. Newborn girls, for example, are 4 to 6 weeks advanced in skeletal age and remain at about 125 percent of male skeletal age until they are sexually mature (Tanner, 1961). Differences in skeletal or sexual maturation are obviously not direct correlates of sex differences in brain maturation or behavior. The enormous regional variations of normal central nervous system maturation make it very unlikely, in fact, that any single behavioral or physiological measure would adequately reflect "brain maturation." On a more limited scale, however, Witelson and Pallie (1973), for example, have shown that selected structures of the left cerebral hemisphere, associated with language processing, are morphologically more mature in newborn girls than boys. From a comparison of sex differences in behavioral outcomes among children with early left- or right-temporal lobe seizures, Taylor (1969) also concluded that the left cerebral hemisphere matures earlier in girls than boys. Finally, Goldman and her associates (1974) observed significant sex differences in behavioral outcome of infant mammals after surgical lesions of the frontal lobes, from which they could infer that there are also sex differences in the cerebral maturation of nonhuman mammals.

The study of human differential abilities provides more extensive but less direct evidence for sex differences in the maturation of cortical functions. Infant girls as a group attain verbal fluency earlier than boys of the same chronological age, and they retain this developmental advantage until adolescence (Garai and Sheinfeld, 1968). Girls perform better than boys of the same chronological age on tasks requiring verbal fluency or speed and accuracy on automatized motor skills (Broverman et al., 1968; Wolff and Hurwitz, 1976). Whether such behavioral sex differences are "real" or experimental artifacts, and if real, whether they are biologically or culturally determined, remain issues which are actively debated (Maccoby and Jacklin, 1974). Any assessment about the merits of this debate must, however, take into account that behavioral sex differences are very sensitive to developmental effects, some differences decreasing as children approach puberty, others not appearing until the onset of the adolescent growth spurt, still others increasing from childhood into adult life. Many inconsistencies in the experimental literature on behavioral sex differences would probably be resolved if maturational factors and developmental changes were systematically considered in the evaluation of research findings.

The biological basis of behavioral sex differences is demonstrated more clearly on performance measures less confounded by cultural factors. They are reflected, for example, in the separate age norms given for boys and girls on the Lincoln-Oseretsky Test of Motor Maturity (Sloan, 1955), the Bender Visual Gestalt Test (Koppitz, 1964), and many other standardized testing procedures (Garai and Sheinfeld, 1968). Childhood behavioral disorders associated with neurological immaturity rather than neurotic conflict or brain damage, such as language and reading retardation, specific learning disability, minimal cerebral dysfunction, motor immaturity or developmental clumsiness, hyperkinesis and attentional disorders, occur 4 to 10 times as often in boys as girls (Bentzen, 1963; Eisenberg, 1966; Singer, Westphal, and Niswander, 1968). A number of the so-called "soft" signs of pediatric neurology are considered normal when they occur in young children and to have diagnostic significance only after a certain age. These disappear significantly later in normal boys than in normal girls, and also persist longer in children with minimal brain dysfunction, specific learning disability and hyperkinesis than in normal children (Connoly and Stratton, 1968; Hurwitz et al., 1972; Wolff and Hurwitz, 1976).

Clinical and experimental evidence converges on the conclusion that specific biological parameters modify the development of normal and abnormal behavioral sex differences, and that girls as a group are "programmed" to mature earlier than boys. Yet, no comprehensive psychological theory of development has systematically incorporated biological mechanisms that might determine such differences in its explanatory formulations. I suggest that our knowledge about maturational mechanisms that contribute to behavioral sex differences is sufficient at present, so that studies that "control for" sex differences by limiting the study sample, or that "control for" maturational rate by grouping children according to chronological age, are likely to miss a crucial determinant of behavioral development.

The indisputable fact of sexual dimorphism does not, however, justify the assumption that males and females constitute dichotomous behavioral types. In cross-sectional and longitudinal follow-up studies, Ljung (1965) and Kohen-Raz (1974) have demonstrated that even within sex the timing of the adolescent growth spurt is closely related to rapid changes of performance on mental tests. Early-maturing girls tend to have a slight but distinct advantage over late-maturing girls of the same chronological age on academic achievement tests (Tanner, 1961); also, Epstein (1974) has reported significant within-sex correlations between rapid changes of physical brain growth and intellectual performance during adolescence.

Waber (1976) has added a new perspective to our understanding about the origins of behavioral sex differences by comparing differential ability profiles in normal early- and late-maturing boys and girls. Early-maturing boys were found to show a typical "female" profile of differential abilities, late-maturing girls a "male" profile. Group differences in cognition and perception, which are generally attributed to sexual dimorphisms, may therefore be explained, at least in part, by the fact that girls as a group mature earlier than boys.

The better performance of boys and men than that of girls and women on most tasks of spatial visualization, of mental rotation for spatial relations, and of visual or tactile pattern recognition (MacFarlane-Smith, 1964; Witelson, 1974) suggests, moreover, that a "general growth factor" is not sufficient to explain the biological contribution to behavioral sex differences. The male advantage on most tests of spatial ability does not become evident until shortly before puberty, but in isolated cases it has been demonstrated as early as 6 years of age (Witelson, 1974). Co-twin variance studies (Bock and Vandenberg, 1968) and family pedigree studies (Hartlage, 1970) have shown that, in addition to maturation, genetic factors contribute directly to sex differences in spatial ability, probably as a sex-linked recessive trait. Moreover, Broverman and his colleagues (1968) have shown that circulating gonadal steroids systematically influence the cognitive style of adults, and that the same endocrine substance has a qualitatively different effect on males and females. We may conclude that no single mechanism adequately explains biologically determined sex differences in behavior, and that such differences are probably the residues of an interaction among genetic, direct hormonal and maturational factors, which exercise their effect in different ways at different stages in ontogenesis.

The relation between brain maturation and behavioral outcome is obviously complex, and susceptible to continuous developmental transformations. Any systematic endeavor to examine how maturation, independent of chronological age, codetermines behavioral development must therefore apply psychological measures that are based on knowledge of brain functions from a developmental perspective. Recent advances in neuropsychology have provided one set of analytic tools which, if properly modified for the study of children, should enable us to investigate the maturation of human behavior in a precise manner. Although most of our information about human brain-behavior relations comes from clinical observations on adult patients with localized cerebral lesions, the concordance between such information and the data from experimental studies on normal children and adults justifies the conclusion that the two cerebral hemispheres are inherently programmed to mediate qualitatively different psychological functions, and that hemispheric specialization does not differ quantitatively in children and adults.

Among right-handed individuals, the left hemisphere is "programmed" to process discrete language functions, the sequential features of nonverbal arrays (Carmon and Nachsohn, 1972), and the serial organization of motor actions (Carmon, 1971; Milner, 1972; Ingram, 1975; Wolff and Hurwitz, 1976). In contrast, the right cerebral hemisphere is preferentially organized for processing information in which visual-spatial features, pattern recognition, and the instantaneous apperception of spatial relations are prominent. The bewildering array of discrete psychological tasks with a partial hemispheric lateralization that has been collated by experimental neuropsychology in recent years has motivated classification of lateralized functions in terms of functional "modes" rather than specific psychological tasks. Thus, the left cerebral hemisphere has been characterized as processing by focal, analytic, or serial strategies, and the right hemisphere as extracting information by the diffuse, holistic, gestalt mode or by strategies of "parallel" processing (Taylor, 1932; Semmes, 1968; Cohen, 1973). Such characterizations are only a rough approximation of actual conditions, but they have the heuristic advantage of grouping a large number of heterogeneous psychological tasks under a few formal rules, and of directing research efforts to a functional analysis of brain mechanisms.

The study of adult patients with hemispheric disconnections (Sperry, 1964; Nebes, 1974) confirms some of the earlier hypotheses about the modal characteristics of hemispheric lateralization, but at the same time reveals that many important psychological functions can either not be carried out or are performed at a lower level of efficiency when the corpus callosum of the mature brain is surgically severed. The intact cerebral cortex seems to have a qualitatively different functional organization than can be inferred from a consideration of the functions performed by each intact hemisphere alone. A comparison of performance deficits in children with a congenital absence of the corpus callosum (Saul and Gott, 1973) and in adult patients with surgical callosectomies further suggests that the developmental analysis of interhemispheric cooperation and competition may be as critical to our understanding of brain-behavior relations as the study of lateralized functions per se.

The contribution of interhemispheric connections to the development of behavior remains a matter of debate. Kimura (1961) and Sparks and Geschwind (1968) proposed a structural model in which information is transferred between two intrinsically lateralized hemispheres. Kinsbourne (1975) has argued for a less static model which assumes a bilateral representation of functions, a suppression of function in the "nondominant" hemisphere by way of the corpus callosum, and a fluctuating distribution of attention across the hemispheres according to task demands. Verbal stimuli, for example, bias attention toward the left hemisphere, whereas certain classes of nonverbal stimuli shift attention to the right hemisphere, and this distribution of attention influences the mode in which information will be processed. When task demands exceed the capacity of either hemisphere, a "time-sharing arrangement" or activation of both hemispheres may be put into effect (Kinsbourne, 1975). Callosectomized patients, unlike normal subjects, cannot simultaneously perform two tasks that are "lateralized" to the same hemisphere, although they can perform each task separately (Kreuter, Kinsbourne, and Trevarthen, 1972). Similarly, when normal children are asked to perform two tasks simultaneously, such as tapping a finger as fast as they can while repeating a familiar verbal passage, the verbal task interferes more with performance of the right than the left hand (Kinsbourne and McMurray, 1975). The "overload" phenomenon is markedly reduced in adults, but it can be demonstrated by increasing the difficulty of the verbal task. The extent of overload by two competing tasks also differs significantly between left- and right-handed adults (Hicks, 1975).

We have examined the development of interhemispheric interactions from a somewhat different perspective by asking children to entrain on the beat of a metronome and to maintain that beat as precisely as possible, after the metronome is turned off, by tapping with one hand alone or the two hands in alternation. Right-handed girls show greater temporal precision as well as an earlier onset of manual asymmetry favoring the right hand. Sex differences as well as manual asymmetries on this task disappear between 11 and 13 years of age (Wolff and Hurwitz, 1976). On a more complex unimanual motor task, however, adults show the same right-hand advantage and females tap with greater precision than males (Wolff, Hurwitz, and Moss, in press). Thus asymmetries in motor performance, as well as sex differences in degrees of asymmetry, persist into adult life, even when the performance measures by which asymmetry was demonstrated in childhood no longer show either sex differences or manual asymmetries.

When we compared the tapping performance of each hand tapping alone and in alternation with the other hand, the better performance of the right hand (on single-hand trials) increased the steadiness in performance of the left hand on alternating-hand trials, whereas the poorer performance of the left hand (on single-hand trials) interfered with the temporal precision of the right hand on alternating-hand trials. Such interaction effects decreased in ontogenesis, but could be demonstrated in adults on a more difficult motor task. Children identified as poor readers in the third grade tapped with significantly less stability than average readers on both the single- and alternating-hand trials (Wolff and Hurwitz, in preparation). In contrast, 11- to 13-year-old boys with severe reading retardation tapped as well as normal readers on the single-hand trials, but their performance on alternating-hand trials was significantly inferior to that of controls (Badian and Wolff, in press). Thus, the older retarded readers continued to show a deficit on motor tasks that presumably require interhemispheric coordination (Lawrence and Kuypers, 1965), but performed as well as normal readers when the same task could be mediated by one hemisphere (Denckla, 1974).

In recently completed studies, we have compared the performance on unimanual and bimanual tapping tasks in normal right- and left-handed males and females, adding a secondary verbal interference task as one experimental variation. A detailed presentation of results would go beyond the purposes of this chapter, especially as we have no adequate explanation at present for many of the complex interactions. A preliminary analysis of data is consistent with reports by others that the verbal task interferes significantly more with performance of the right than of the left hand on *single-hand trials*, but also indicates that the verbal task interferes significantly more with performance of the left than of the right hand on *alternating-hand trials*. A simple "overload" hypothesis is therefore inadequate to account for the interhemispheric interactions under different conditions of "hemispheric loading." The degree and direction of interference by a verbal task were also found to vary systematically with sex and hand preference; moreover, the sex-by-hand preference interactions changed as a function of age. Three biological variables that are generally assumed to influence the organization of behavior —maturational age, sex, and hand preference—thus appear to influence the performance of normal adults on psychological tasks requiring interhemispheric cooperation (Marshall, 1973; McGlone and Davidson, 1973).

I would like to consider one clinical example which may illustrate how developmental neuropsychology may help to explain the behavioral disturbances of children who come to the attention of the child psychiatrist. Many children, particularly boys, who are of normal or superior intelligence and free of organic or major neurosensory deficits, have had the advantage of adequate schooling, and were well motivated to learn (at least in the early school years), fall increasingly behind in academic work because they do not acquire the necessary reading skills. DeHirsch, Jansky, and Langford (1966), Bakker (1972), and Satz and his colleagues (1971, 1973, 1974) tested Orton's maturational-lag hypothesis for specific reading retardation in longitudinal follow-up designs. The nonreading measures of psychological performance administered in kindergarten were found to be efficient predictors of later reading retardation. Although the kindergarten predictors were no longer discriminative at the time the reading deficiency became manifest 1 to 2 years later, more differentiated psychological measures again discriminated between groups. Such findings suggest that specific reading retardation involves more than the inability to read, that the impairment of performance in children with reading retardation reflects a maturational delay which can be compensated in ontogenesis, and that the underlying maturational delay can later be demonstrated on more advanced performance measures.

Noting striking surface similarities in the performance profiles of children with specific reading retardation and adult patients with localized lesions of the left hemisphere, Satz further hypothesized that maturational delay in reading retardation may be confined to left-hemisphere-dependent functions. Many children with specific reading retardation, for example, have a history of developmental language retardation, even when they speak normally at the time of school entry (Ingram, 1970); many are delayed in lateralization of function for language processing (Zurif and Carson, 1970; Lake and Bryden, 1976); and many show a specific impairment on the temporal organization of symbolic elements (Bakker, 1972). The hypothesis that reading retardation is associated with a maturational delay of left-hemisphere functions would be consistent with many clinical and experimental observations indicating that retarded readers are specifically deficient in the serial ordering of verbal and nonverbal elements ("left-hemisphere" functions), whereas many of the same children are as proficient as normal readers on tasks of spatial visualization or pattern perception ("right-hemisphere" functions) (Eisenson, 1966; Doehring, 1968; Bakker, 1972; Ingram, 1975). Since the academic skills that determine success in the elementary schools depend almost entirely on functions preferentially processed by the left hemisphere (Crinella, Beck, and Robinson, 1971), it should not be surprising that healthy and intelligent, but late-maturing, children are at great risk of school failure.

The maturational-lag hypothesis has not been critically tested to determine whether maturational delay is entirely susceptible to developmental "catchup." Since many intelligent adults who had severe reading handicaps as children never achieve reading fluency despite extensive remedial tutoring (Perlo and Rok, 1971), one might, in fact, conclude either that remedial tutoring is useless or that specific reading retardation is caused by irreversible lesions of the central nervous system. However, if our earlier speculation is correct that local variations in maturational rate have far-reaching effects on the overall organization of behavioral development, one might expect to encounter irreversible variations in the styles of adaptation or preferred modes of processing, together with reversible deficits on discrete performance measures.

In terms of the concrete example presented, we can now suggest some guidelines by which the clinical syndromes of children may be examined from a psychobiological perspective:

1. The influences of maturational rate on behavioral development, independent of chronological age, are as crucial for our understanding of psychological development as are the influences of differential experience.

2. Somatic growth proceeds by linear or curvilinear pathways. Regional variations in brain growth, on the other hand, result in a continuous qualitative restructuring of part-whole relations that will be reflected in behavioral development as discontinuous periods of rapid acceleration, quiescence, and "learning dips." These in turn will vary with the age of the organism and the differential functions being examined. Assuming that somatic growth and brain maturation are causally related, the nature of their interaction will therefore of necessity be complex and not demonstrable by simple correlations of parallel growth rates.

3. Sex differences in maturational rate are apparent not only for somatic growth but also for psychological development—particularly the development of functions associated with hemispheric lateralization and interhemispheric cooperation.

4. Many behavioral disturbances that come to the attention of the child psychiatrist occur with far higher frequency in boys than in girls and are probably influenced to a major extent by specific maturational factors. Thus, the higher incidence of behavioral disturbances in males may be caused, at least in part, by their relatively slower maturation.

5. The profile of impaired functions in specific reading retardation suggests that the syndrome is associated with a selective delay of functions mediated by the left hemisphere, and of functions requiring cooperation between the two cerebral hemispheres.

6. Maturational delay may result in specific performance deficits that will be compensated in development; it may also be associated with qualitative variations in behavioral organization which remain stable characteristics of the individual. These need not constitute behavioral deficits in any biologically meaningful sense, but may be labeled as deviant in a social context that equates the normal with the average.

If I have been successful in demonstrating a functional relation between variations of maturational rate and developmental profiles, the demonstration would in no way imply a direct causal relation between biology and specific clinical syndromes. Reading retardation, for example, may become a clinical, psychiatrically relevant syndrome when industrialized society expects its children not only to read, but also to read at a particular chronological age; or when educational policy equates intellectual competence with performance on tasks that are processed selectively by the left hemisphere. The severe emotional stresses inflicted on retarded readers are obviously not a consequence of biology, but the result of society's impatience with, or indifference to, normal biological variations in rates or styles of mental development. The excessive reliance on chronological age as the independent variable in developmnt must therefore be held responsible for the unnecessary suffering of biologically healthy children who may be slower than their peers, but who, like the tortoise, might have won the race in a more supportive environment. Since child psychiatrists neither can, nor should, interfere with maturational rate, their essential contribution to primary prevention in this example may be to protect children against society's biologically unsound demands that children should conform to the bell-shaped curve, and to inform parents, teachers, and colleagues about the inherent strength conferred on any society when it encourages individual variations.

REFERENCES

BADIAN, N., and WOLFF, P. H. Motor sequencing skills in boys with learning disabilities. *Cortex*, in press.

BAKKER, D. J. 1972. *Temporal Order in Disturbed Reading*. Rotterdam: Rotterdam University Press.

BENTZEN, F. 1963. Sex ratios in learning and behavior disorders. *Am. J. Orthopsychiatry*, 33:92-98.

BOCK, R. D., and VANDENBERG, S. G. 1968. Components of heritable variation in mental test scores. In S. G. Vandenberg (ed.), *Progress in Human Behavior Genetics*. Baltimore: Johns Hopkins University Press.

BROVERMAN, D. M., KLAIBER, E. L., KOBAYASKI, Y., and VOGEL, W. 1968. Roles of activation and inhibition in sex differences in cognitive abilities. *Psychol. Rev.*, 75:23-50.

CARMON, H. 1971. Sequential motor performance in patients with unilateral cerebral lesions. *Neuropsychologia*, 9:445-450.

CARMON, H., and NACHSOHN, I. 1972. Effect of unilateral brain damage on perceptions of temporal order. *Cortex*, 8:410-418.

CHESS, S. 1971. Autism in children with congenital rubella. *J. Autism Child. Schizo.*, 1:33-37.

COHEN, G. 1973. Hemispheric differences in serial versus parallel processing. *J. Exp. Psychol.*, 97:349-356.

CONNOLY, K., and STRATTON, P. 1968. Developmental changes in associated movements. *Dev. Med. Child Neurol.*, 10:49-56.

CRAVIOTO, J., DeLICARDIE, E. R., and BIRCH, H. G. 1966. Nutrition, growth and neurointegrative development: An experimental and ecologic study. *Pediatrics*, 38:319-372.

CRINELLA, F. M., BECK, F. W., and ROBINSON, J. W. 1971. Unilateral dominance is not related to neuropsychological integrity. *Child Dev.*, 42:2033-2054.

DE HIRSCH, K., JANSKY, J. J., and LANGFORD, W. S. 1966. *Predicting Reading Failure: A Preliminary Study*. New York: Harper & Row.

DENCKLA, M. B. 1974. Development of speed in repetitive and successive finger movements in normal children. *Dev. Med. Child Neurol.*, 15:635-645.

DOBBING, J. 1968. Vulnerable periods in the developing brain. In A. N. Dawson and J. Dobbing (eds.), *Applied Neurochemistry*, pp. 287-316. Oxford: Blackwell.

DOBBING, J., and SANDS, J. 1971. Vulnerability of the developing brain: The effect of nutritional growth retardation on the timing of the brain growth spurt. *Biol. Neonate*, 19:363-378.

DOEHRING, D. G. 1968. *Patterns of Impairment in Specific Reading Disability*. Bloomington, Indiana: Indiana University Press.

EISENBERG, L. 1966. The epidemiology of reading retardation and a program for preventive intervention. In J. Morey (ed.), *The Disabled Reader*. Baltimore: Johns Hopkins University Press.

EISENSON, J. 1966. Perceptual disturbances in children with central nervous system dysfunctions, and implications for language development. *Disord. Communic.* 1:21-32.

EPSTEIN, H. T. 1974. Phrenoblysis. Special brain and mind growth periods. II. Human mental development. *Dev. Psychobiol.* 7:217-224.

GARAI, J. E., and SHEINFELD, A. 1968. Sex differences in mental and behavioral traits. *Genet. Psychol. Monogr.*, 77:169-299.

GOLDMAN, P. S., CRAWFORD, H. T., STOKES, L., GALKINS, T. W., and ROSVOLD, H. E. 1974. Sex-dependent behavioral effects and cerebral cortical lesions in the developing Rhesus monkey. *Science*, 186:540-542.

HARTLAGE, L. C. 1970. Sex-linked inheritance of spatial ability. *Percep. Mot. Skills*, 31:610.

HICKS, R. E. 1975. Intrahemispheric response competition between vocal and unimanual performance in normal adult males. *J. Comp. Physiol. Psychol.*, 80:50-60.

HURWITZ, I., BIBACE, R. M. A., WOLFF, P. H., and ROWBOTHAM, B. 1972. Neuropsychological function of normal boys, delinquent boys, and boys with learning problems. *Percept. Mot. Skills*, 35:387-394.

INGRAM, D. 1975. Motor asymmetries in young children. *Neuropsychologia*, 13:95-102.

INGRAM, T. T. S. 1970. The nature of dyslexia. In F. A. Young and D. B. Lindsley (eds.), *Early Experience and Visual Information Processing in Perceptual and Reading Disorders*, pp. 403-444. Washington, D.C.: National Academy of Science.

KIMURA, D. 1961. Cerebral dominance and the perceptions of verbal stimuli. *Can. Psychol.* 15:166-171.

KINSBOURNE, M. 1975. Lateral interactions in the brain. In M. Kinsbourne and W. L. Smith (eds.), *Hemispheric Disconnections in Cerebral Function*, pp. 239-259. Springfield, Ill.: Thomas.

KINSBOURNE, M., and McMURRAY, J. 1975. The effect of cerebral dominance on time sharing between speaking and tapping by preschool children. *Child Dev.*, 46: 240-242.

KOHEN-RAZ, R. 1974. Physical maturation and mental growth in preadolescence and puberty. *J. Child Psychol. Psychiatry*, 15:199-213.

KOPPITZ, E. M. 1964. *The Bender Gestalt Test for Children*. New York: Grune & Stratton.

KREUTER, C., KINSBOURNE, M., and TREVARTHEN, C. 1972. Are disconnected cerebral hemispheres independent channels? A preliminary study of the effects of unilateral loading on bilateral finger tapping. *Neuropsychologia*, 10:453-461.

LAKE, D. A., and BRYDEN, M. P. 1976. Handedness and sex differences in hemispheric asymmetry. *Brain Language*, 3:266-282.

LAWRENCE, D. G., and KUYPERS, H. G. J. M. 1965. Pyramidal and nonpyramidal pathways in monkeys: Anatomical and functional correlations. *Science*, 148:973-975.

LJUNG, B. O. 1965. The adolescent spurt in mental growth. *Stockholm Studies in Educational Psychology*, vol. 8. Stockholm: Almqvist & Wikseil.

MACCOBY, E. E., and JACKLIN, C. N. 1974. *The Psychology of Sex Differences*. Stanford, California: Stanford University Press.

MACFARLANE-SMITH, I. 1964. *Spatial Ability*. London: University of London Press.

MARSHALL, J. C. 1973. Some problems and paradoxes associated with recent accounts of hemispheric specialization. *Neuropsychologia*, 31:463-470.

McGLONE, J., and DAVIDSON, W. 1973. The relation between cerebral speech laterality and spatial ability with special reference to sex and hand preference. *Neuropsychologia*, 11:105-113.

McKHANN, G. M., COYLE, P. K., and BENJAMINS, J. A. 1973. Nutrition and brain development. *Res. Publ. Assoc. Res. Nerv. Ment. Dis.* 51:10-22.

MILNER, B. 1972. Interhemispheric differences and psychological processes in man. *Br. Med. Bull.* 27:272-277.

NEBES, R. D. 1974. Hemispheric specialization in commissurotomized man. *Psychol. Bull.*, 81:1-14.

ORNITZ, E. M., and RITVO, E. R. 1976. The syndrome of autism: A critical review. *Am. J. Psychiatry*, 133:609-621.

PERLO, V. F., and ROK, E. T. 1971. Developmental dyslexia in adults. *Neurology*, 21:1231.

PURPURA, D. P. 1973. Analysis of morphological developmental processes in mammalian brain. *Res. Publ. Assoc. Res. Nerv. Ment. Dis.* 51:79-112.

RAKIC, P., and YAKOVLEV, P. I. 1968. Development of the corpus callosum and cavum septi in man. *J. Comp. Neurol.* 132:45-72.

RICCIUTI, H. N. 1973. Malnutrition and psychological development. *Res. Publ. Assoc. Res. Nerv. Ment. Dis.* 51:63-77.

SATZ, P., RARDIN, D., and ROSS, J. 1971. An evaluation of a theory of developmental dyslexia. *Child Dev.*, 42:2009-2021.

SATZ, P., and VANNOSTRAND, G. K. 1973. Developmental dyslexia: An evaluation of a theory. In P. Satz and J. J. Ross (eds.), *The Disabled Learner*, pp. 212-248. Rotterdam: Rotterdam University Press.

SATZ, P., FRIEL, J., and RUDEGAIR, I. 1974. Differential changes in the acquisition of developmental skills in children who later become dyslexic. In D. Stein, J. J. Rosen and N. Butters (eds.), *Recovery of Function*, pp. 175-202. New York: Academic Press.

SAUL, R. E., and GOTT, P. S. 1973. Compensatory mechanisms in agenesis of the corpus callosum. 25th annual meeting, American Academy of Neurology, Boston.

SEMMES, J. 1968. Hemispheric specialization: A possible clue to mechanism. *Neuropsychologia*, 6:11-26.

SINGER, J. E., WESTPHAL, M., and NISWANDER, K. R. 1968. Sex differences in the incidence of neonatal abnormalities and abnormal performance in early childhood. *Child Dev.*, 39:103-112.

SLOAN, W. 1955. The Lincoln-Oseretsky motor development scale. *Genet. Psychol. Monogr.*, 51:183-251.

SPARKS, R., and GESCHWIND, N. 1968. Dichotic listening in man after section of neocortical commissures. *Cortex*, 4:3-16.

SPERRY, D. W. 1964. The great cerebral commissure. *Sci. Am.*, 210:42-52.

TANNER, J. M. 1961. *Education and Physical Growth*. London: London University Press.

TANNER, J. M. 1970. Physical growth. In P. H. Mussen (ed.), *Carmichael's Manual of Child Psychology*, pp. 77-155. New York: Wiley.

TAYLOR, D. C. 1969. Differential rates of cerebral maturation between sexes and between hemispheres. *Lancet*, 2:140-142.

TAYLOR, J. (ed.). 1932. *Selected Writings of John Hughlings Jackson*, vol. 2. London: Hodden & Stoughten.

TREVARTHEN, C. 1974. Cerebral embryology and the split brain. In M. Kinsbourne and W. L. Smith (eds.), *Hemispheric Disconnections in Cerebral Function*, pp. 208-236. Springfield, Illinois: Thomas.

WABER, D. P. 1976. Sex differences in cognition: A function of maturation rate? *Science*, 192:572-573.

WHITE, S. R. 1970. Some general outlines of the matrix of developmental changes between 5-7 years. *Bulletin of the Orton Society*, 20:41-57.

WITELSON, S. F., and PALLIE, W. 1973. Left hemisphere specialization for language in the newborn. *Brain*, 96:641-646.

WITELSON, S. F. 1974. Hemispheric specialization for linguistic and nonlinguistic tactual perception using a dichotic stimulation technique. *Cortex*, 10:3-17.

WOHLWILL, J. 1973. *The Study of Behavioral Development*. New York: Academic Press.

WOLFF, P. H. 1970a. What we must and must not teach our children from what we know about cognitive theory. In P. H. Wolff and R. MacKeith (eds.), *Planning for Better Learning*, pp. 7-19. London: Heinemann.

WOLFF, P. H. 1970b. Motor development and holotelencephaly. In R. Robinson (ed.), *Brain and Early Behavior*, pp. 139-169. London: Academic Press.

WOLFF, P. H., and HURWITZ, I. 1973. Functional implications of the minimal brain syndrome. *Semin. Psychiatry*, 5:105-116.

WOLFF, P. H., and HURWITZ, I. 1976. Sex differences in finger tapping: A developmental study. *Neuropsychologia*, 14:35-41.

WOLFF, P. H., HURWITZ, I., and Moss, H. Serial organization of motor skills in left- and right-handed adults. *Neuropsychologia*, in press.

YAKOVLEV, P. I., and LECOURS, A. R. 1967. The myelinogenetic cycles of regional maturation of the brain. In A. Minkowski (ed.), *Regional Development of the Brain in Early Life*, pp. 3-70. Oxford: Blackwell.

ZURIF, E. B., and CARSON, G. 1970. Dyslexia in relation to cerebral dominance and temporal analysis. *Neuropsychologia*, 8:351-358.

2

Genetics and Behavioral Development

GERALD E. McCLEARN, Ph.D.

My principal aim is to present a perspective of modern genetics, particularly as it pertains to understanding the sources of human individuality and variability. I hope also to provide enough data to be persuasive that this perspective is not only applicable, but worthy of broader application in the study of behavioral development.

Galton's neat alliterative phrase, "nature-nurture," has made it all too easy to perpetuate the dichotomous view that characteristics are determined either by hereditary or by environmental factors. That the either-or dichotomy should be replaced by a both-and formulation is easily seen by *reductio ad absurdum*: An organism without heredity or an organism without an environment cannot exist; it will have no traits whatsoever. It is meaningful, however, to ask about the relative contributions of individual differences in genetic endowment and in present and past environmental circumstances to measured differences in some particular trait. Formally, this proposition may be expressed (with some simplifying assumptions—see Falconer, 1960) as $V_P = V_G + V_E$, where V_P represents the total phenotypic variance (or measured variance), V_G represents the variance due to genetic differences, and V_E represents the variance due to environmental differences.

Perhaps the best way to understand this model of the sources of variability in a trait is in terms of a simple example. In the first column of Table 1, each of 16 individuals is characterized by a

TABLE 1

A Model of Polygenic Inheritance with Environmental Influence

Genotype	Genotypic Value	Environmental Effect I	Phenotype I	Environmental Effect II	Phenotype II
AABB	4	—1	3	—2	2
AABb	3	+1	4	+2	5
AABb	3	0	3	0	3
AaBB	3	0	3	0	3
AaBB	3	0	3	0	3
AAbb	2	+1	3	+2	4
AaBb	2	—1	1	—2	0
AaBb	2	+1	3	+2	4
AaBb	2	+2	4	+4	6
AaBb	2	0	2	0	2
aaBB	2	—2	0	—4	—2
Aabb	1	0	1	0	1
Aabb	1	+1	2	+2	3
aaBb	1	—1	0	—2	—1
aaBb	1	—1	0	—2	—1
aabb	0	0	0	0	0
	$V_G=1$	$V_E=1$	$V_P=2$	$V_E=4$	$V_P=5$
		"heritability"=.50		"heritability"=.20	

statement of its *genotype* (genetic makeup) with respect to two different genes. Each of these genes exists in two alternate forms: The first can be either A or a, and the second can be B or b. (The 16 individuals shown in the table would be the idealized results of the cross of an AaBb male with an AaBb female.) For simplicity, let us assume that each of these genes influences the same trait in such a fashion that a small letter adds nothing, while a big letter in the genotype adds one unit. Thus, the AABB individual has a value of 4, and the aabb individual has a value of 0. If these values are plotted, the distribution shown at the top of Figure 1 is obtained. The mean

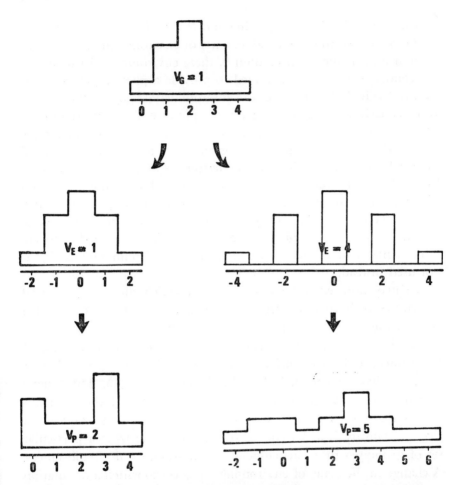

FIGURE 1. A simple model of genetic, environmental, and phenotypic variance.

of this distribution is 2 and its variance (which is all genetic variance) is 1, as shown at the bottom of Table 1.

Let us consider environmental influences that can either add to or subtract from the value determined by the genotype. Furthermore, let us assume that these environmental effects are binomially distributed as shown in Figure 1 and that they are assigned randomly to the different individuals in such a fashion that there is no correla-

tion between the genotypic value and the environmental one. One of the many possible such assignments of environments is shown in column 3 of Table 1. In column 4, these environmental values and the genotypic values are summed to provide a phenotypic value for each individual. The mean of the environmental values is 0 and their variance is 1. The mean of the phenotypic values is 2 and their variance is 2. It may be seen that, of the total variance of the phenotypic distribution (which is portrayed graphically at the bottom left of Figure 1), one-half is due to genetic sources of variability and one-half is due to environmental sources. In a broad sense, the proportion of the total phenotypic variance that is ascribable to genetic sources is called *heritability*. It is only an historical accident that the inverse index, the proportion of the total phenotypic variance due to environmental sources (which we might call "environmentability"), is not used instead.

We may now examine a situation in which the environmental determinants have a relatively larger influence. By doubling the effect, either positive or negative, of each environmental factor, and proceeding as before, the phenotypic array in column 6 of Table 1 is obtained. This distribution is shown at the bottom right of Figure 1. It also has a mean of 2, but the variance is now 5. The genetic variance has remained the same (i.e., 1), and the heritability in this case is therefore .20. This example illustrates the important point that heritability is a descriptive statistic, characterizing a particular set of genotypes in a particular set of environmental circumstances. A change in the array of environmental forces to which a population is exposed can result in a change in heritability. This model emphasizes that both genetic and environmental sources may contribute to the variability displayed in a trait; it does not require that one choose a side, and one side only, in the nature-nurture controversy.

The model just presented is, of course, greatly oversimplified. For example, many more than two different genes may influence a particular behavior. (It should also be noted that the model becomes a simple Mendelian one when only a single gene is involved.) Various elaborations are necessary to deal with correlations between genotype and environment and with complex interactions among genes and between genes and environment.

Given such analytical models, what is the nature of the empirical evidence that genes do, in fact, influence behavior? Evidence can be cited from research on both animals and human beings. In the animal literature, most compelling results have been obtained by the comparison of inbred strains of mice. The process of inbreeding, or of mating relatives, over a sufficiently long period of time leads to a situation in which all of the animals within a strain are, for all practical purposes, identical genetically. If two or more different inbred strains are reared and tested in the same laboratory environment, then any differences that exist among them may be attributed to differences in the genotypes that have come to exist among the strains as they developed. Such comparisons have shown wide differences among strains in activity levels of various kinds, in learning of a variety of tasks, in memory processes, in aggressiveness, in hoarding behavior, in alcohol preference, and in numerous other traits. Figure 2 illustrates the kinds of results obtained in this line of research. The upper part of the figure shows activity scores of three different groups, all lumped together. A very substantial variability in activity level is displayed. When the groups are separated, it can be seen that a large part of that variability is attributable to a between-strains component and therefore to genotypic differences. Also noteworthy is the variability that remains within each group, attributable to environmental differences among the animals within the groups. Once again, we see the importance of both genetic and environmental forces. The genotypic effects are so powerful that the most active of the A strain is less active than the least active of the C57BL strain. On the other hand, environmental variability remaining in the carefully controlled experimental situation is sufficiently great to make one C57BL animal only half as active as another C57BL.

Another technique used in animal behavioral genetics is that of selective breeding. Very briefly, beginning with a genetically heterogeneous foundation population, animals displaying a high extreme for the trait of interest are mated together, as are animals displaying low extremes of the same trait. Two lines are thus established, and

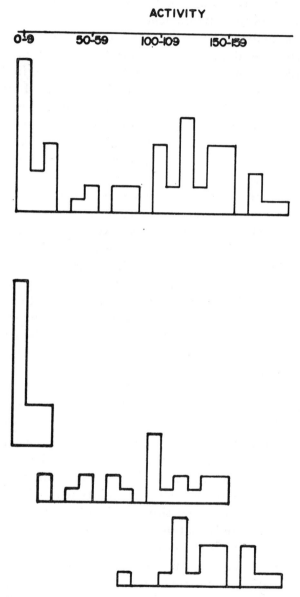

FIGURE 2.   Activity scores of C57BL, F1, A, and combined groups (from bottom to top).

in successive generations the highest are mated with the highest in the high line and the lowest mated with the lowest in the low line. Such a technique enabled Tryon (1940), in his classical work, to generate maze-bright and maze-dull rats. Subsequently, researchers have reported successful selective breeding for a variety of behavioral attributes, including activity level, aggression, alcohol acceptance, learning ability, and several other traits in mice and rats.

Although there is no human equivalent of the inbred strain or selected line, evidence of genetic influence on behavior in human-kind is available from a variety of sources. The example of sensory deficits due to single genes has long been known. Colorblindness, for instance, has been recognized as a sex-linked inherited character-istic since about 1910. More recently, the interesting difference among people in ability to taste phenylthiocarbamide (PTC) has been shown to be determined by a single gene. While the ability or inability to taste PTC has not yet been related to "important" psy-chological variables (and may never be so linked), this phenomenon does serve as an important heuristic in suggesting that we may differ substantially in our sensory and perceptual processing functions and that important contributions to these differences may be made by our genotypes.

Single genes have also been shown to determine various types of mental retardation. The classic example, of course, is phenylketonu-ria. Investigations of the mechanisms through which the gene exerts its influence (the nature of the enzymic defect and the metabolic consequences) have made possible systematic attempts at early iden-tification and rational therapy. Single-gene influences on mental re-tardation also include other conditions involving abnormal amino acid metabolism and conditions related to disorders of lipid metabol-ism and carbohydrate metabolism.

Another type of evidence dealing with anomalies of behavior has been provided by studies of chromosomal abnormalities. The best-known example is probably that of Down's syndrome (formerly de-scribed as mongolism), which is due to the presence of extra material from a particular small chromosome (number 21). Absence of part of another chromosome (number 5) gives rise to the *cri du chat* syndrome of mental retardation. Absence of chromosomal material in the case of the sex chromosomes, where the individual has only a single X chromosome, gives rise to the well-known Turner's syndrome, which includes not only symptoms of lack of sexual development but also a specific cognitive deficit in dealing with spatial relations.

The principal methods which have been used in investigating genetic influences on individual differences within a normal range of variability have been twin studies, studies of family resemblance, and adoption studies. The twin studies, in which resemblance of identical twins is compared to resemblance of fraternal twins, have provided evidence consistent with the hypothesis of genetic influence on a variety of behavioral traits, including IQ, personality characteristics, and susceptibility to psychoses. Similarly, in studies of the resemblance of offspring to parents, a series of investigations has explored the same range of behaviors, with results generally consistent with those of the twin research. One example of a recent large-scale study of familial resemblance is the Hawaii study on genetic and environmental bases of cognitive functioning (DeFries et al., 1976). The results presented in Table 2 are based on measures of resemblance of offspring to parents in some 700 families on a variety of paper-and-pencil tests and on four factors derived by multivariate analysis. It must be emphasized that human family studies do not have the precision of control possible in laboratory studies with animals. In interpreting these results, the possibility of a correlation between genotype and environment must be kept in mind. That is, individuals with genotypes making for extreme expression of one of these characteristics, either in the upward or the downward direction, may experience environments conducive to development of the trait in the same direction. Given that this possibility exists, the regression coefficients provided in Table 2 must be accepted only as upper-limit estimates of heritability. These estimates do strongly suggest, however, that different components of intellectual functioning may have different relative contributions of genotype and environment.

A particularly powerful approach in human behavioral genetic research is the adoption study. Early studies of this sort suffered from

TABLE 2

Regression of Mid-Child on Mid-Parent (± Standard Error) for Cognitive Tests and Factor Scores

	Regression Coefficient
TESTS	
Vocabulary	.68±.04
Visual Memory (immediate)	.26±.05
Things	.55±.04
Mental Rotations	.48±.05
Subtraction and Multiplication	.40±.04
"Lines and Dots" (Elithorn Mazes)	.25±.05
Word Beginnings and Endings	.56±.04
Card Rotations	.53±.04
Visual Memory (delayed)	.53±.04
Pedigrees	.74±.04
Hidden Patterns	.47±.05
Paper Form Board	.63±.04
Number Comparisons	.48±.04
Social Perception	.39±.05
Progressive Matrices	.59±.04
FACTORS	
Verbal	.65±.04
Spatial	.61±.04
Perceptual Speed	.46±.04
Visual Memory	.44±.05

the effects of late adoption, selective placement, and other problems, but recent procedures have reduced the difficulties considerably. The work of Heston (1970) and of Rosenthal (1971) and Rosenthal et al. (1971) has provided compelling evidence as to the existence of genetic factors in schizophrenia. Thus, the results of adoption studies agree with the findings of twin and family studies in suggesting that genetic influence on behavior is ubiquitous.

Of particular interest and relevance to studies of children are observations that the full information content of the genotype is not unleashed, so to speak, at the moment of conception. It is becoming

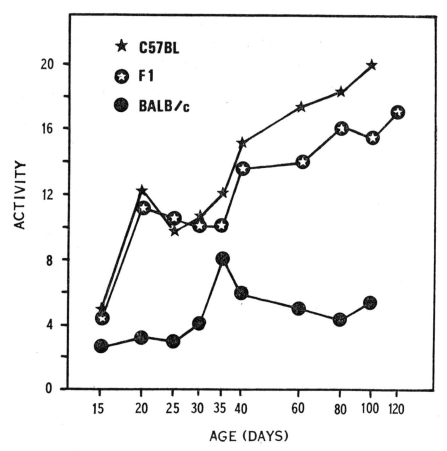

FIGURE 3. Activity scores of C57BL, Fl, and BALB mice as a function of age.

increasingly clear that different genes are "turned on" in different tissues and that, in any particular tissue, different genes may be called into play at different stages in the developmental process.

Several tactics have been employed in studying the genetics of behavioral development in animals. One approach has been simply to describe changes as a function of age in different genetic groups. Dixon and DeFries (1968), for example, examined changes with age in open-field activity of the inbred C57BL and BALB strains and their F1 hybrid offspring. The results are shown in Figure 3. It can be seen that there was essentially no change with age in the BALB strain and a striking increase in activity of the C57BL animals, while the hybrids were like their more active parent at early ages and came to be somewhat more intermediate with increasing age. Another approach has been to examine strain differences in response to various interventions during infancy. A good example is the work of Lindzey and Winston (1962) in which "gentling" had a favorable effect on the performance of C57BL mice in a maze, but had practically no effect on C3H mice. A particularly dramatic outcome was obtained by Weir and DeFries (1964), who found that mild stress administered to pregnant mice had the effect of increasing activity of the grown young in the BALB strain, while activity was decreased in the C57BL strain.

In human research, genetic influence on behavioral development has been illustrated by Honzik's (1957) observations showing an age-related increase in resemblance of offspring to biological parents but not to adoptive parents on a measure of intellectual functioning. Wilson's (1972) demonstration of correlated spurts and lags in cognitive development in young monozygotic twins and the finding by Jarvik et al. (1972) that twins retained similarities during their declining years point to genetic influence on behavioral development throughout the total life span.

It is probably fair to say that only a bare beginning has been made in the study of human developmental behavioral genetics. Indeed, even the use of animal models has been minimal to date. The work that has been done, however, offers a strong promise that future investigations in this area of research will yield significant new insights into human individuality and the developmental processes through which it is attained.

REFERENCES

DeFries, J. C., Ashton, G. C., Johnson, R. C., Kuse, A. R., McClearn, G. E., Mi, M. P., Rashad, M. N., Vandenberg, S. G., and Wilson, J. R. 1976. Parent-offspring resemblance for specific cognitive abilities in two ethnic groups. *Nature*, 261: 131-133.

DIXON, L. K., and DeFRIES, J. C. 1968. Development of open-field behavior in mice: Effects of age and experience. *Dev. Psychobiol.,* 1:100-107.

FALCONER, D. S. 1960. *Introduction to Quantitative Genetics.* New York: Ronald Press.

HESTON, L. L. 1970. The genetics of schizophrenic and schizoid disease. *Science,* 167:249-256.

HONZIK, M. P. 1957. Developmental studies of parent-child resemblance in intelligence. *Child Dev.,* 28:215-228.

JARVIK, L. F., BLUM, J. E., and VARMA, A. O. 1972. Genetic components and intellectual functioning during senescence: A 20-year study of aging twins. *Behav. Genet.,* 2:159-171.

LINDZEY, G., and WINSTON, H. 1962. Maze learning and effect of pretraining in inbred strains of mice. *J. Comp. Physiol. Psychol.,* 55:748-752.

ROSENTHAL, D. 1971. Two adoption studies of heredity in the schizophrenic disorders. In M. Bleuler and J. Angst (eds.), *The Origin of Schizophrenia,* pp. 21-34. Bern: Verlag Hans Huber.

ROSENTHAL, D., WENDER, P. H., KETY, S. S., WELNER, J., and OSTERGAARD, L. 1971. The adopted-away offspring of schizophrenics. *Am. J. Psychiatry,* 128:307-311.

TRYON, R. C. 1940. Genetic differences in maze-learning ability in rats. *Yearbook of the National Society for the Study of Education,* 39 (1):111-119.

WEIR, M. W., and DeFRIES, J. C. 1964. Prenatal maternal influence on behavior in mice: Evidence of a genetic basis. *J. Comp. Physiol. Psychol.,* 58:412-417.

WILSON, R. S. 1972. Twins: Early mental development. *Science,* 175:914-917.

Part II
RISK RESEARCH AND PRIMARY PREVENTION

3

The Infant at Risk–Assessment and Implications for Intervention

DAVID B. EAGLE, M.D.
and
T. BERRY BRAZELTON, M.D.

As we continue to make progress in the area of early intervention, it becomes increasingly important to be able to evaluate infants at risk. The problems of at-risk infants are compounded by environments that are not adjusted to their special needs. Premature and (minimally) brain-damaged infants seem to be less able to compensate in disorganized, depriving environments than are well-equipped neonates (Greenberg, 1971). Because the central nervous system of these infants is either immature or compromised as the result of mechanical and/or chemical injury, these infants are under more stress than full-term, healthy newborns. A depriving environment is an additional force that prevents the kind of integration of central nervous system (CNS) mechanisms necessary for the recovery and plasticity in maturation of an already vulnerable CNS. Our research indicates that even mildly SGA (small for gestational age) infants may be included in this vulnerable group.

Quiet, undemanding infants do not elicit necessary caretaking from already overstressed parents, and in poverty-ridden cultures, like those that can be found in Guatemala and Mexico (Cravioto, DeLicardie,

This work was supported by the R. W. Johnson and Carnegie Foundations.

and Birch, 1966; Klein, Habicht, and Yarbrough, 1971), these infants are selected by their neonatal behavior for kwashiorkor and marasmus. They are quiet babies, perhaps because of malnourishment in utero, and since they do not make their needs known, they are left alone. Hyperkinetic, hypersensitive neonates may produce a desperation in parents that causes the parents to overreact, thus reinforcing the infant's problems. These babies have difficulty controlling their own reactions to inner and environmental stimuli, and they demand frequent interactions with their parents. Their behavior patterns are irregular and therefore confusing to the parents, who often feel incompetent and guilty as a result. This, in turn, is detrimental to the attachment process.

Parents of children admitted to the wards of Children's Hospital in Boston for clinical syndromes such as failure to thrive (FTT), child abuse, neglect, ingestion of poisons, and recurrent accidents are often successful parents of other children. They mention an inability to understand their child from the beginning, and say that the infant's earliest reactions to them were different from those of their other children. These infants and environments need to be identified as early as possible so that supportive intervention can begin. Parents who feel that they are to blame for a difficult infant must be assured that their infant is *normal*, but *different* from their other children.

The job of the neonate is to adapt to the change from intrauterine to extrauterine environment, which involves a myriad of internal and external factors. Part of this job is to elicit the caretaking that will supply the necessities of infancy. Infants have many capabilities to do this; at-risk infants have a harder job. Unfavorable environments make the job harder, even for well-organized infants. We need more sophisticated methods for assessing neonates and for predicting their contribution to the likelihood of failure of the environment-infant interaction. We also need to be able to assess at-risk environments. With better techniques for assessing strengths and weaknesses in infants and the environments to which they will be exposed, we might better understand the mechanisms of failure in development that result in some of the syndromes referred to earlier. Understanding the infant and the problems that it will present to the family may enhance our value as supporting figures as the parents adjust to a difficult infant. If we can help organize environments and if we can help parents recognize that they are not solely responsible for their infant's behavior, we will increase the probability of their success in coping with a difficult situation.

Present Methods of Assessment

Apgar Score and Neurological Exam

The commonly used examinations to assess risk in infancy—the Apgar Score (1953), pediatric and neurological tests—are able to detect gross abnormalities, but they have not been as successful in discovering mild dysfunction of the CNS during the neonatal period. Drage et al. (1966) found a fourfold increase in neurological abnormalities in year-old infants with Apgars of 0 to 5 compared to those with Apgars of 7 to 10 at five minutes. But only 4.3 percent of those with low Apgars demonstrated gross abnormalities at seven years, and there was a poor correlation between Apgar scores and mild CNS dysfunctions. The Apgar score reflects the infant's ability to make the immediate adjustment to the stress of the birth process, but it does not predict later recovery or decompensation. Its five categories—color, respiration, heart rate, tone, and response to aversive stimuli—measure the functions necessary to sustain life. The score is influenced by any perinatal event: hypoxia, drugs, anesthesia, prolonged labor, Caesarian section, etc., but since it is done in the first 15 minutes after delivery only, it basically measures the immediate capacity of the neonate for an alarm reaction. The depression that may occur later and may represent the baby's depleted resources is not predicted by the Apgar score. If more sensitive tests are used along with it, however, the Apgar score may help predict future areas of difficulty. For example, Lewis et al. (1967) studied visual attentiveness at 3, 9, and 13 months of age in babies with Apgars of 7 to 10 at one minute. Lewis's group was able to differentiate between babies with scores of 7 to 9 and those with scores of 10 in their capacity to respond to complex visual tasks.

The concept that the newborn functions only at a brainstem level of organization (Peiper, 1963) led to stereotyped neurological examinations which assessed reflex behavior with an oversimplified positive-negative (all or none) approach. More recent neurological examinations no longer make this assumption (Prechtl and Beintema, 1964). It is now believed that higher brain centers modify responses through partial inhibition or facilitation in the neonate, and that the intact function of the CNS can be determined by a *qualitative* assessment of responses in the neonatal period. Brain-damaged infants may have reflex responses, but these may be exaggerated or depressed, stereotyped or obligatory; the quality of these responses is different from that of the graded ones seen in an intact baby. Infants who are functioning mostly on a midbrain level, such as those with anencephaly, show little evidence of habituation or grading of repeated responses until exhaustion causes extinction.

The Prechtl examination (Prechtl and Beintema, 1964) gives credit to this capacity on the part of the neonate. It stresses the state of arousal within which each set of evaluations is made and points to the significant qualitative differences that are present in the different states. It is sensitive to the modifying function of the higher brain centers on reflex activity. This exam and those of Thomas and Ajuriagueiria (1949), Saint Anne Dargassies (1966) and Parmelee and Michaelis (1971) stress muscle tone at rest, in active and passive movements, and asymmetrical differences, in predicting minor and major CNS residual damage.

These examinations record discrete reflex and postural behavior and not the more complicated responses to social stimulation that may reflect a higher order of organization and integration of physiological and neurological systems in the neonate. Gross abnormalities are evaluated, but not milder dysfunctions. The exams concentrate on the neonate's capacity to organize his or her responses to disturbing stimuli, but they miss the infant's alerting responses to positive stimuli.

For example, a neurological exam of visual functioning consists of eliciting pupillary closure to bright light, assessing extra-ocular movements, nystagmus, doll's eye reflex, and fundus. But the infant is capable of more sophisticated visual performances. The neonate can habituate the initial blink and startle responses to a bright light. The response to a moving object consists of widening of the pupils and eyelids, facial softening, inhibition of generalized body movements, and coordinated tracking movements of eyes with head movements of 180 degrees (Tronick and Clanton, 1971). Some neonates "search" for the object if it is lost during tracking. The infant can make decisions about stimuli, which can be quantified by duration of attention (Kessen, Haith, and Salapatek, 1970). These responses are observable in a well-organized neonate and decreased or absent in stressed infants. Hack, Mostow, and Miranda (1976) suggest that the human brain may be capable of waking states by as early as 31 to 32 weeks of gestation and may be able to process sensory information. Studying the development of attention in premature infants, they found that behaviors associated with visual fixation increased steadily from 31 to 36 weeks of gestational age. More attention to these kinds of complex behaviors will allow professionals to make more accurate assessments of the intactness of the newborn.

Another example is motor integrity. The neurological exam assesses reflexes and tone, but pays little attention to the infant's capacity to perform more complicated maneuvers like bringing hand to mouth with head turning to meet the fist, then insertion and sucking. The fact that this movement is used by an upset infant to maintain control is ignored. The smoothness and range of movements shown by an infant during quiet, alert states as opposed to his less controlled behavior when he is upset might give the observer a range of behavior that could predict the infant's capacity to organize his neuromotor system in alert as well as in defensive, upset states.

The neonatal intensive-care nursery is an environment in which the type of assessment just discussed could be applied clinically for preventive and supportive purposes. It is the type of environment in which one is likely to find an infant in an upset, disturbed state many times during a 24-hour period. The high-risk nursery is a chaotic, disorganizing place when looked at in terms of the physiological needs of the newborn, especially a sick newborn. Sleep-wake cycles are disrupted because the lights are never off, and procedures are undertaken at any time. The noise level in an isolette is above the tolerable range. Feedings are on schedule rather than on demand. Contact with adults, especially parents, is haphazard. All of this means that an infant's cues for letting his or her needs be known are rarely noticed unless the cue is apnea, seizures, or cardiac arrest. Very little of what happens to the infant depends on the infant's behavior. If an observer could document how well and in what way an infant organizes his or her nervous system to maintain control in the face of this onslaught, the observer might be able to predict whether that infant will make it, at least in the nursery. Such an assessment would also help the staff caring for the infant to become more aware of that infant as an individual living entity and to structure the environment appropriately. The information would also help parents relate to their baby and therefore foster attachment.

Parmelee and Michaelis (1971) stressed the importance of repeated neurological exams, believing that the best predictor of long-term outcome is the speed/curve of recovery of impaired function during the first few days or weeks of life. Delay in recovery of complex functions may reflect an insult from which the brain cannot recover without permanent impairment. These authors urged closer and more frequent attention to complex neonatal behavior as predictive of infants at risk. This behavior includes observations of *sleep states and alertness,* habituation, and integrated motor activities like sucking and swallowing, and creeping when prone.

Before describing the behavioral exam designed to elicit the organized responses and capabilities of the neonate, it is important to mention that many other factors need to be considered. Clinical assessment of the amniotic fluid, placenta, cord, and cord blood is vital to any prediction of risk in the neonate. These tissues may reflect deprivation and predict future problems. For example, Klein, Habicht, and Yarbrough (1971) in Guatemala found placental weight in poor and protein-deficient groups 10 percent less than normal. The infants were underweight and undersized for gestational age. The protein deficiency is associated with a gamma-globulin level in the cord blood 10 times that of a U.S. control group, suggesting a synergism between lowered protein intake and high levels of infection which endanger the developing fetus.

In addition, it is important to assess the neonate for signs of prematurity and/or dysmaturity. Small-for-date and premature infants face more risk than do well-nourished full-term infants (Brazelton, 1973a). Their functioning on any form of neonatal assessment is also altered by these conditions. Differentiation between short- and long-term deprivation must be made. The tools developed by Lubchenko et al. (1963) and Dubowitz, Dubowitz, and Goldberg (1970) help assess the maturity of the neonate. More refined techniques such as nerve-conduction velocity tests, electroencephalograms, and quantitative ratios of REM to deep-sleep cycles are substantiating evidence for the stage of CNS maturation.

Behavioral Examination

With all these tools available for assessment, there still remained the need for a more sophisticated evaluation scale to document the neonate's integrative processes, the use of state behavior, and the response to various kinds of positive (social) stimuli. The Brazelton Neonatal Assessment Scale (Brazelton, 1973b) was designed for this purpose. Since the infant's reactions to all stimuli depend on the ongoing state, any interpretation must be made with this in mind. The infant's use of state to maintain control of his reactions to environmental and internal stimuli is an important mechanism and reflects the potential for organization. State does not need to be considered an interfering variable; it is major evidence of CNS organization. The exam tracks state changes, lability, and direction over the course of the exam. The variability of state points to the capacities for self-organization. An infant who manifests all states of consciousness and who can change state appropriately with or without environmental stimulation indicates a greater capacity for organization and control than an infant who cannot demonstrate this range of behavior or who is "locked into" a state in an obligatory way. Understanding the concept of state (Prechtl and Beintema, 1964) makes it easier to understand an infant's behavior.

The awake states are:

1. *Deep sleep* with regular breathing, eyes closed and without movements, and no spontaneous activity except startles or jerky movements at irregular intervals; external stimuli produce startles with some delay; suppression of startles is rapid, and state changes are less likely than from other states.

2. *Light sleep* with eyes closed; rapid eye movements under lids. Low activity level. Movements smoother than in state 1. State changes possible with external stimuli. Respirations irregular, sucking movements occur on and off.

1. *Drowsy* with eyes opening and closing or partially or fully open with glazed look. Generalized motor activity may be seen and respirations are fairly regular, but more frequent and more shallow than in sleep states. State changes frequently after stimulation.

2. *Quiet alert* with little movement but eyes bright and clear. Eyes seem to focus on source of stimulation.
The sleep states are:

3. *Fussing*—similar to quiet alert with mild, agitated vocalizations.

4. *Crying* with intense, generalized motor activity and continuous crying.

One example of the influence of state on behavior will be given here. If a rattle is shaken when an infant is in a drowsy state, the infant may startle, slow down movement, and then either change state and become more sleepy, or remain drowsy. The infant in a quiet alert state may pause in respiration or movement, widen the eyes, and then begin to search for the source of the sound. An examination based on knowledge of state will be more accurate and physiologically valid than if state is not taken into consideration.

The ability to use stimulation also measures the availability for social interaction. An infant who can come to an alert state with stimulation from an examiner or parent, or can likewise be consoled, shows the capacity to organize in order to interact with the environment. The ability to self-quiet points to organization *not* dependent on the environment. Which type of stimulation a particular infant will use depends on that infant's unique personality and helps to establish his or her individuality in the eyes of the caretaker.

The Brazelton Neonatal Behavioral Exam tests for neurological adequacy with 20 reflex measures and 26 behavioral responses to environmental stimuli, including the kind of interpersonal stimuli parents use in their handling of the infant. The exam uses a graded series of procedures—talking, hand on belly, restraint, holding, and rocking—designed to soothe and alert the infant. The responses to animate stimuli (e.g., voice and face) and to inanimate stimuli (e.g., rattle, bell, red ball, white light, temperature change) are assessed. Vigor and attentional excitement are measured, as are motor activity, tone, and autonomic responses with state change.

The exam is best given as late as possible on the third day of life, after the period of depression and disorganization following the initial alert state immediately after delivery. This third period may be the best single predictor of individual potential function and the results seem to correlate well with those of the 30-day retest. The shape of the curve made by several exams may be the most important assessment of the intactness of the infant's ability to integrate CNS and other physiological recovery mechanisms. It is especially important when there have been compromising insults during labor and delivery.

The behavioral items are listed in Table 1.

We believe that the behavioral items are tapping important evidences of cortical control and responsiveness, even in the neonatal period. The neonate's capacity to manage and overcome the physiological demands of this adjustment period in order to attend to, differentiate, and habituate to the complex stimuli of an examiner's maneuvers may be an important predictor of future CNS organization. The curve of recovery during the first neonatal weeks is more significant than the midbrain responses detectable in routine neurological exams.

The predictive value of the behavioral exam was compared with that of the neurological exam by using seven-year outcomes as part

TABLE 1

Behavioral Items of Brazelton Neonatal Behavioral Assessment Scale*

Response decrement to repeated visual stimuli
Response decrement to a repeated auditory stimuli
Response decrement to pinprick
Orienting responses to inanimate visual and auditory stimuli
Orienting responses to the examiner's face and voice
Quality and duration of alert periods
General muscle tone—in resting and in response to being handled (passive and active)
Motor maturity
Traction responses as he/she is pulled to sit
Responses to being cuddled by the examiner
Defensive reactions to a cloth over his/her face
Consolability with intervention by examiner
Attempts to console self and control state behavior
Rapidity of buildup to crying state
Peak of excitement and his/her capacity to control himself
Irritability during the exam
General assessment of kind and degree of activity
Tremulousness
Amount of startling
Lability of skin color (measuring autonomic lability)
Lability of states during entire exam
Hand-to-mouth activity

* from Brazelton, 1973b.

of the National Institutes of Health Collaborative Study (#BP 2372) done at Boston Lying-In Hospital for Women. The two exams were similar in their capability for detecting abnormal infants. The neurological exam correctly diagnosed 13 of the 15 neonates who later turned out to be abnormal, and the Brazelton assessment diagnosed 12 of the 15. None of the children was still labeled suspect at outcome. There were striking differences, however, in the discriminative ability of the two exams. The neurological exam classified 43 infants as "suspect/abnormal," and 13 turned out to be abnormal. Thirty neonates misdiagnosed as being "suspect/abnormal" later turned out to be "normal." This is a false-alarm rate of 80 percent. Thus, the neurological exam obtained its success rate of 87 percent by misclassifying a large percentage of "normal" infants. In contrast, the Brazelton scale diagnosed 21 neonates as "suspect/abnormal," and 12 of these were abnormal at outcome. Nine were misdiagnosed, a false-alarm rate of 24 percent. The Brazelton scale achieved its success rate of 80 percent by detecting abnormal neonates without mislabeling as many normal infants. How can the differences be accounted for? The Brazelton exam found the same abnormalities as did the neurological assessment, but it weighed them against the infant's ability to perform integrated acts that pointed to a higher level of CNS functioning, such as alerting, orientation, and self-quieting, as described above. Even with abnormalities of functioning, some infants classified as suspect neurologically could be classified as normal by a Brazelton exam.

The differences may also be related to differences in the way the tests are done. The Brazelton exam is designed to uncover an infant's *optimal performance* over the 20 to 30 minutes it takes to do the assessment. Assessments are made twice and the curve of recovery is noted. The examiner is flexible in the way that he or she tries to bring out a response. The examiner comforts and supports an infant's attempts to maintain motor and state control, and in this way enhances the infant's state of alertness. Because of this, many disorganized infants can demonstrate the ability to organize and control their alert state. This indicates future capabilities after they have recovered from the neonatal period. These are especially important for temporarily disorganized infants, like those whose mothers have had large doses of drugs during delivery.

What is the effect of mislabeling on these infants and their parents? We have no data, but such a self-fulfilling prophecy (Merton, 1948) might be expected to have harmful effects on parental expectations (Rosenthal and Rosnow, 1969).

What are the other uses of the scale? The exam has been used in cross-cultural studies, with prematures and SGA infants, to document behavioral correlates of intrauterine protein depletion, and to assess the influence of medication given to the mothers during labor and delivery. The scale's assessment of capabilities for higher-order functioning may also have advantages for modifying the hospital and home environment for infants. Infants of narcotics-addicted mothers were found to be difficult to deal with because of their irritability and jerkiness, but it was discovered that restraining the movements of the infants and having a quiet, softly lighted environment helped bring them to a more organized state. The hospital staff was better able to care for these infants after the changes were made. When a clearer picture is obtained about the strengths and weaknesses of a particular infant or group of infants, the environment can then be made more appropriately responsive to their developmental needs.

By uncovering some of the strengths and weaknesses of a particular infant, we become more aware of that infant as an individual. We become aware of what the infant is offering to the environment and the things to which the parents might react. With this information, we may be able to help foster attachment, anticipate problems, and decrease anxiety by saying to the parents that we are interested, and that we see what they see: the good as well as the not so good, or the spectrum of normality. We (Brazelton, Eagle, and J. M. Cupoli) are studying infants who are small for gestational age and are finding that they tend to be irregular in their rhythms, to be very sensitive to stimulation, and to have difficulty organizing. They are hard to reach socially, which is disturbing to their parents. Because these infants are usually called "normal" by the obstetrician and pediatrician, the parents blame themselves for having a difficult infant. If we can identify these infants early and discover their particular strengths and capacities, we can relate this to their parents and make the situation more realistic and less guilt-producing. We demonstrate the behavioral exam to parents, and in this way they see what we see.

One assessment that should be developed is the evaluation of infant-mother or infant-parent interactions. Bowlby (1969) suggests that the mother may have attachment responses that are triggered by the neonate's behavior. Klaus and Kennell (1970) described the kinds of initial contacts mothers make with their newborn infants and the distortions in this behavior when the mother is distressed by abnormalities in the baby. Eye-to-eye contact, touching, handling, and nursing behavior may be assessed for predicting her ability to relate to the new baby. Changes in these behaviors over time indicate recovery or nonrecovery of capacity to attach to the baby by mothers who have been depressed or unable to function optimally by having produced an infant at risk. The opportunity for observing this process is best in the lying-in period. It is vital that we provide infants at risk with the best possible environment to foster their capacity to recover and integrate any intact mechanism for development.

REFERENCES

APGAR, V. A. 1953. A proposal for a new method of evaluation of the newborn infant. *Current Researches in Anesthesia and Analgesia*, 32:260-267.

BOWLBY, J. 1969. *Attachment and Loss*, vol. 1. *Attachment*. New York: Basic Books.

BRAZELTON, T. B. 1973a. Assessment of the infant at risk. *Clin. Obstet. Gynecol.* 16: 361-375.

BRAZELTON, T. B. 1973b. Neonatal behavioral assessment scale. In *Clinics in Developmental Medicine*, No. 50. London: Spastic International Medical Monographs. Philadelphia: Lippincott.

CRAVIOTO, J., DELICARDIE, E. R., and BIRCH, H. G. 1966. Nutrition, growth and neuro-integrative development: An experimental and ecologic study. *Pediatrics*, 38 (2) Part 2:319-372.

DRAGE, J. S., KENNEDY, C., BERENDES, H., SCHWAB, K., and WEISS, W. 1966. The Apgar score as an index of infant morbidity. A report from the collaborative study of cerebral palsy. *Dev. Med. Child Neurol.*, 8:141-148.

DUBOWITZ, L. M., DUBOWITZ, V., and GOLDBERG, G. L. 1970. Clinical assessment of gestational age in the newborn infant. *J. Pediatr.*, 77:1-10.

GREENBERG, N. H. 1971. A comparison of infant-mother interactional behavior in infants with atypical behavior and normal infants. In *Exceptional Infant*, vol. 2. New York: Brunner/Mazel.

HACK, M., MOSTOW, A., and MIRANDA, S. 1976. Development of attention in preterm infants. *Pediatrics*, 58:669-674.

KESSEN, W., HAITH, M., and SALAPATEK, P. 1970. Infancy. In P. H. Mussen (ed.), *Manual of Child Psychology*, vol. 1, pp. 287-445. New York: Wiley.

KLAUS, M. H., and KENNELL, J. H. 1970. Mothers separated from their newborn infants. *Pediatr. Clin. North Am.* 17:1015-1037.

KLEIN, R. E., HABICHT, J. P., and YARBROUGH, C. 1971. *Effect of Protein Calorie Malnutrition on Mental Development*. Institute of Nutrition of Central America and Panama (Incap) Publication No. 1-571.

LEWIS, M., BARTELS, B., CAMPBELL, H., and GOLDBERG, S. 1967. Individual differences in attention. *Am. J. Dis. Child.*, 113:461-465.

LUBCHENKO, L. O., HANSMAN, C., DRESSLER, M., and BOYD, E. 1963. Intrauterine growth estimated from liveborn, birthweight data at 24 to 42 weeks gestation. *Pediatrics*, 32:793-800.

MERTON, R. K. 1948. The self-fulfilling prophecy. *Antioch Review*, 8:193-210.

PARMELEE, A. H., and MICHAELIS, R. 1971. Neurological examination of the newborn. In *Exceptional Infant*, vol. 2. New York: Brunner/Mazel.

Peiper, A. 1963. *Cerebral Function in Infancy and Childhood*. New York: Consultants Bureau.

Prechtl, H., and Beintema, O. 1964. *The Neurological Examination of the Full Term Newborn Infant*. Little Club Clinics in Developmental Medicine, No. 12. London: Heineman.

Rosenthal, R., and Rosnow, R. L. 1969. *Artifact in Behavioral Research*. New York: Academic Press.

Saint Anne Dargassies, S. 1966. Neurological maturation of the premature infant of 28 to 41 weeks gestational age. In F. T. Falkner (ed.), *Human Development*. Philadelphia: Saunders.

Thomas, A., and Ajuriagueiria, J. 1949. *Étude Semiologique du Tonus Musculaire*. Paris: Médicales Flammarion.

Tronick, E., and Clanton, C. 1971. Infant looking patterns. *Vision Research*, 11:1479-1486.

4

Observations on Research with Children at Risk for Child and Adult Psychopathology

NORMAN GARMEZY, Ph.D.

Introduction

Risk research implies a developmental orientation to psychopathology reflecting two underlying assumptions: first, that there are identifiable individuals who have heightened potential for later disorder; second, that such potential typically is actuated by stressful biological, psychological, sociocultural, or familial factors. There is a continuity between this orientation and the view held by many mental health professionals that the early years of a disturbed adult's life had a critical import for the behavior pathology that followed.

It is not the orientation that has posed problems, but, rather, the methodology that has been used traditionally to validate the premise. Rooted in a historical commitment to retrospection for retracing antecedent events, psychiatry has focused inappropriately on adult recall for recording the critical contents of those early years. One can always look back on history with a sense of omniscience that bears at best a faint analogy to wisdom, but history provides an awareness of the shortcomings in psychiatry's traditional developmental orientation to psychopathology. Psychiatrists recognized early

The preparation of this paper was facilitated by a Research Career Award (NIMH), MH-K6-14, and a grant from the Schizophrenia Research Program, The Supreme Council 33° A.'.A.'. of the Scottish Rite, Northern Masonic Jurisdiction, USA.

the power of antecedents rooted in childhood for understanding disordered behavior. However, they paved the way for errors of content and interpretation by remaining overly dependent upon a reconstructive methodology that required disordered adults or their family members and friends to recall past events and relationships in an effort to understand a disordered present.

Why this primary allegiance to the faulty process of recall? One can account for the support of an unreliable methodology by noting that in the pursuit of a *structured* or *descriptive* account of behavior disorder, or in the choice of a more *dynamically attuned* orientation, historical tradition came down affirmatively on the side of adult study. Both Kraepelin, brilliant taxonomer, and Freud, dynamic psychiatry's great architect, shared as a common focus the study of disordered adults. But, as I recently noted:

> ... for Kraepelin, intent on describing *ongoing* psychiatric states, the here-and-now behavior of the disordered patient was the appropriate object of inquiry. For Freud, that same here-and-now behavior as a mechanism for unlocking the past was fraught with unsuspected traps. It is well to note that even genius can be trapped, as witness the slow dawning of awareness for Freud that those numerous incestuous themes from the lips of maiden ladies, to whom he had listened with such care, were all too often constructed out of whole cloth. Only genius can salvage such an error and come forth with an even more illuminating conceptualization than the power of *actualized* incest, namely that the true power lies in the wish that fathers the unacceptable thought and that must then take disguised form for a partial actualization to take place (Garmezy, 1977, p. 2).

Unfortunately, what must be carefully noted is the important distinction between the role of the therapist versus that of the etiologist. The former works with distortion, using it to provide the patient with a more accurate perception and understanding of the present; by contrast, for the etiologist, distortion of true past events can block understanding of the present and inevitably produce a set of cognitive culs-de-sac for those who seek the origins of disorder.

Simply stated, retrospections, however faulty, do serve a therapeutic purpose, but what serves the purpose of treatment too often prevents effective etiological theorizing.

There is a social value to be added here as well. Not only can retrospection do a disservice to the cause of etiological understanding, but if treated with exaggerated respect, reconstructive accountings can bring misery to many innocent and blameless persons. One need only consider the climate of the 50s in which therapists saw fit to label mothers of adult schizophrenic patients as "schizophrenogenic" or to assign the "refrigerator" appelation to parents of autistic children to realize the dangers of a too ready set to infer the past from observations made in the present.

What was ignored in those two clinical examples was the importance of the *bidirection of effects* in studies of the socialization of children (Bell, 1968; Lewis and Rosenblum, 1974). In a volume on *The Effect of the Infant on Its Caregiver,* a title which reflects the newer orientation, Bell (1974) has written:

> Recent reviews of research on the effect of parent practices or techniques . . . now uniformly recommend caution in interpreting correlations between parent and child characteristics in a unidirectional fashion, and some even go further, offering substantive interpretations of the correlations in terms of the effects of children on parents (p. 1).

The importance of this newer orientation for studying disordered children can be illustrated by reference to a number of recent areas of research.

CHILD ABUSE AND RISK RESEARCH

To illustrate the application of Bell's viewpoint, one can turn to an important area of risk research—child abuse. So aberrant is the phenomenon of child battering, and so distasteful is it to clinicians and researchers alike, that there is a powerful tendency to focus exclusively on the deviant parent to explain pathological caretaking. Abusing parents have been described as overly dependent, lacking in impulse control, and immature, qualities so widely evident in our society as to provide few insights into those who batter and cripple their offsprings (Steele and Pollock, 1971). Immaturity in parents is clearly far more prevalent than the incidence rates for child abuse in the nation. A backward look to the early lives of abusing parents has also generated a statement marked by stereotypic overgeneralization: Battering parents, we are told, were once battered children. To appreciate the potenital etiologic error in this statement, one must perceive that images of continuity are inevitable if one works backward from an end point of pathology in an effort to understand the roots of disorder. Were the process to be reversed, the number of assigned false positives would be legion. Let me illustrate this point with an anecdote.

Because of an unfortunate worldwide newspaper story in which my current research interest in "invulnerable" children was prematurely revealed, I received many letters from adults around the nation who had themselves been battered children and who, in adulthood, were leading productive lives. Many wrote of their positive response to the concept of "invulnerability," describing their lives in some detail, in which a powerful component was their determination to see to it that their children would lead far happier lives than they had known. Despite their earlier trauma, all had rejected its repetition in their own families.

Freud (1920) has provided an insightful observation on the preconditions for etiological error:

> So long as we trace the development from its final stage backwards, the connection appears continuous, and we feel we have gained an insight which is completely satisfactory or even exhaustive. But if we proceed the reverse way, if we start from the premises inferred from the analysis and try to follow these up to the final result, then we no longer get the impression of an inevitable sequence of events which could not be otherwise determined. We notice at once that there might have been another result, and that we might have been just as well able to understand and explain the latter. The synthesis is thus not so satisfactory as the analysis; in other words, from a knowledge of the premises we could not have foretold the nature of the result.

It is very easy to account for this disturbing state of affairs. Even supposing that we thoroughly know the aetiological factors that decide a given result, still we know them only qualitatively, and not in their relative strength. Some of them are so weak as to become suppressed by others, and therefore do not affect the final result. But we never know beforehand which of the determining factors will prove the weaker or the stronger. We only say at the end that those which succeeded must have been the stronger. Hence it is always possible by analysis to recognize the causation with certainty, whereas a prediction of it by synthesis is impossible (pp. 226-227) .

In the light of this insightful analysis of "followback" evaluations, what seems to be the factual evidence that maltreating parents were maltreated children? Jayaratne (1977) seriously questions the data that are available, pointing out the lack of adequate normal control comparison groups to support the presumed relationship and citing Gil's (1970) national study that had revealed that 7 percent of fathers and 14 percent of mothers in the abusing sample had themselves been victims of child abuse in their own childhoods.

Jayaratne concludes:

. . . available data do not substantiate the direct and significant correlation that—according to the generational hypothesis— exists between abuse experience and abusing behavior. It is perhaps too simplistic to argue that innumerable events occurred during the period under consideration (from the time the parents allegedly were abused until the time they were abusing their own children) and that some of these happenings might explain much of the variance. This is nonetheless true, and the simplicity of the explanation belies the complexity of the picture (p. 8) .

Here again is an example of inadequate etiological speculation that has the power to victimize innocent persons through inadvertent labeling based upon such speculation.

If we turn back to Bell's position, the complexity of child abuse would suggest the importance of a transactional view of the parent-child relationship in which aggression is triggered by the interaction of the attributes of abusing parent and abused child. More recent research has been directed toward understanding the stimulus value that a specific child in a family constellation may have for the abusing parent, suggesting that this factor may help to account for the coexistence of battering and nonbattering within many families (Parke and Collmer, 1975; Klein and Stern, 1971).

In describing their psychiatric study of parents who abuse infants and children, Steele and Pollock (1974) have written:

> There is no doubt that the infant, innocently and unwittingly, may contribute to the attack which is unleashed upon him. An infant born as the result of a premaritally conceived pregnancy or who comes as an accident too soon after the birth of a previous child, may be quite unwelcome to the parents and start life under the cloud of being unrewarding and unsatisfying to the parents. Such infants may be perceived as public reminders of sexual transgression or as extra, unwanted burdens rather than need-satisfying objects. An infant may also be seen as "uncooperative" or unsatisfying by having been born a girl when the parents wanted a boy or vice versa. Babies are born with quite different behavioral patterns. Some parents are disappointed when they have a very placid child instead of a hoped-for, more reactive, responsive baby. Other parents are equally distressed by having an active, somewhat aggressive baby who makes up his own mind about things when they had hoped for a very placid, compliant infant. A potent source of difficulty is the situation in which babies are born with some degree, major or minor, of congenital defect, therefore requiring much more medical as well as general attention. Often such infants are fussy, crying, and difficult to comfort and are limited in their ability to respond as a normal, happy baby should. Intercurrent illness may produce a similar picture. Babies born prematurely require much more care and offer less response soon enough to satisfy the parents' needs. . . .
> Thus, it is obvious that characteristics presented by the infant, such as sex, time of birth, health status, and behavior are factors in instigating child abuse (pp. 114-115).

Obviously the issue is not one of assigning blame. But the passage above contains a number of transactional referents that parallel the formulations provided by Thomas, Chess, and Birch (1968) in their volume on *Temperament and Behavior Disorders in Children*. From the standpoint of etiology such findings suggest the importance of considering at least a partially reactive rather than a simple unidirectional etiological model in child abuse.

ATTACHMENT BEHAVIOR AND RISK RESEARCH

Another problem that has inhibited the growth of a true developmental perspective in psychopathology is the adherence to a linear growth model as exemplified by the-child-is-father-of-the-man concept. Children, as Wolff also points out in this volume, are not miniaturized adults passively awaiting maturity. Piaget's seminal contributions make clear that the child moves through stage sequences marked by unique transformations in behavior that reflect increasingly complex patterns of differentiation and organization accompanied by more complexly integrated patterns of cognitive and social maturity and competence.

One can turn away from pathological caretaking to the more positive aspects of attachment behavior and the formation of affectional bonds to note the importance of the quality of the mother-infant bond from an organizational perspective. Deviant variations in patterns of attachment may also provide a significant contribution to later deviant personality formation in some children.

In a recent paper Bowlby (1977) has described the organizational quality of attachment behavior:

> Initially attachment behavior is mediated by responses organized on fairly simple lines. From the end of the first year, it becomes mediated by increasingly sophisticated behavioural systems organized cybernetically and incorporating representational models of the environment and self. These systems are activated by certain conditions and terminated by others. Among activating conditions are strangeness, hunger, fatigue and anything frightening. Terminating conditions include sight or sound of mother-figure and, especially, happy interaction with her. When attachment behaviour is strongly aroused, termination may require touching or clinging to her and/or being cuddled by her.

Conversely, when mother-figure is present or her whereabouts well-known, a child ceases to show attachment behaviour and, instead, explores his environment (pp. 203-204).

The developmental consequences of variations in this basic attachment pattern have recently been studied by Sroufe and his colleagues (Sroufe, in press; Sroufe and Mitchell, in press; Sroufe and Waters, in press).

These investigators have been studying longitudinally the development of emotional responsiveness in children up to age two whose relationships to mother are suggestive of secure vs. insecure attachment bonds. In studies covering the first year of life evidence has accumulated to suggest that a secure attachment relationship has adaptive consequences in other behavioral domains, since it bears a significant relationship to a child's ability at age two to explore and master the inanimate environment, to achieve a concept of an autonomous self, to manifest early signs of social and play competence, cognitive competence in terms of object permanence and exploratory activity, and engagement with unfamiliar persons.

Sroufe notes that unpublished research with Matas reveals security of attachment to be related to "later problem solving style (spirit of engagement, persistence), joy in problem solution, compliance to maternal requests, and other aspects of a dyadic problem solving situation at age two." By contrast, infants who show insecurity of attachment at age 12 months tend later at 24 months to be noncompliant, resistant to contact, avoidant of and aggressive toward the mother. Longitudinal advances to age four are now being planned and will afford a picture of the extent to which the continuity of competence can be adduced from early patterns of infant-mother bonding. It is by such formulations and attendant data that a theoretical framework may be provided for experiments aimed at deriving significant antecedent-consequent relationships between early and stable affectional bonds and subsequent child competence, and between unstable attachment patterns and later incompetence.

For Ainsworth (1972), this is the major reason to explore attachment, for it would appear to provide "fine-grain studies of early intrapersonal interactions and their effect on personality development" (p. 106). For Bowlby (1977), these consequences extend far into adulthood, with pathological early attachments providing the base for disturbed family functioning, differing forms of individual psychopathology, false expectations and beliefs about others, and stereotypic patterns of responsiveness to others, for "whatever representational models of attachment figures and of self an individual builds during his childhood and adolescence, these tend to persist relatively unchanged into and throughout adult life" (p. 209).

In Bowlby's statement lies a suggestion of the complexity necessary to understand the child abuse syndrome. It is to be expected that attachments extending beyond the original caregiver and beyond infancy exercise a marked effect on personality formation. The representation of self is a compound of experiences and interactions that provide a base for self-evaluation and social comparisons. In the complex equation that determines cognitive and social maturity, genetic, constitutional, and temperamental factors also play a significant role in adaptation. Whether the early mother-infant attachment is prototypic of or a heavily weighed precursor to more extended forms of adaptive or disordered behavior can only be determined by systematic longitudinal study in which variations in the adequacy of affectional bonds constitute the independent variable and later competence-patterning is a prominent aspect of the dependent variables to be investigated. Bowlby has suggested that neurotic symptoms, depression, and phobias are often correlated with "disparaging and rejecting" responses to a child's care-eliciting efforts, "discontinuities of parenting," perhaps due to hospitalization or institutionalization, parental incapacity for love, threats of abandonment posing as discipline, and fears of parental death, desertion, or loss.

Such threats, Bowlby asserts, are reflected in the representational models children build of attachment figures and of self and tend to persist into adult life. Other individuals who enter a child's life are assimilated to this internalized model, and behaviors that are in accordance with such models become dominant modes of interacting with others to form the basis for maladaptive life-styles. But here, too, one would anticipate that complexity should prevail and such complexity will only be revealed through a penetrating longitudinal analysis of the development of children in the context of the social milieus they inhabit.

What is particularly interesting about Bowlby's viewpoint is the context it provides for the assertion that to understand disordered development it must be assayed against our knowledge of normal developmental processes. Sir Peter Medawar stated this proposition when he pointed out that "it is not informative to study variations of behavior unless we know beforehand the norm from which the variants depart."

This intimate linkage between normality and aberrance provides some interesting insights into a recent foreword that Piaget wrote to E. J. Anthony's volume on *Explorations in Child Psychiatry* (1975). Here Piaget, who has always disavowed an interest in psychopathological development, refers to "the mechanisms that are implicated in any . . . functional disintegration" and stresses the importance of maintaining an "analytic" approach to the problem of disentangling such mechanisms. Piaget adds:

> However, since there are those who remain normal in situations where others become variously disturbed, the meaning of the disorder to be remedied can be extremely diverse, and in order to grasp it, it is necessary to immerse oneself in the ensemble (of elements involved) at different developmental stages, the order of which is by no means fortuitous but resembles the orderly sequence of stages observed in embryogenesis (pp. vii-viii) .

I find it appealing that Piaget also writes of the development of a new discipline which many now perceive as emerging out of a union of developmental psychology and developmental biology, clinical psychiatry and clinical psychology. Again Piaget:

> To put it briefly, developmental psychologists (including myself . . .) are looking forward with great expectation to the emergence of *developmental psychopathology* as a new discipline still struggling to organize its own relevant field of knowledge.

They are hoping especially that in spite of all the obstacles in the way and the huge amount of creative effort required for the purpose that this science will constitute itself on an interdisciplinary basis as wide as possible and on a common language that helps to unify what is precise and generalizable (p. ix).

CHILDREN AT RISK FOR SEVERE ADULT PSYCHOPATHOLOGY

We are a long way from the goal cited by Piaget and Bowlby but we can identify different types of children who will be of concern to this new breed of developmental psychopathologists. Prominent among these would be children who may, in time, become the victims of some of the most malignant of psychiatric disorders. For the remainder of this chapter I will confine my remarks to risk for adult schizophrenia—an area of research that has engaged my attention in recent years. Our initial interest in children of schizophrenic mothers (as exemplified by the pioneering work of Mednick and Schulsinger [1973]) has been extended not only to these offspring but, with the necessity of securing contrasting risk groups, to the offspring of mothers manifesting depressive and personality disorders, to clinic children who are being treated either for antisocial behavior, or for fearful-avoidant-isolative behaviors, and more recently to hyperactive children. To these groups we have added normal classmates who are peers of the risk children and serve as controls on either a matched or random basis.

Numerous programs of research in recent years have been initiated to study children born of schizophrenic parents on the assumption that such offspring are more predisposed to the subsequent *development* and *maintenance* of schizophrenic pathology in comparison with randomly chosen children drawn from similar communities or neighborhoods.

I have used two key words, *development* and *maintenance*; the first speaks to etiology, the second to prognosis and outcome. The context of development is discriminably different from the maintenance component in that it thrusts the study of risk back to some earlier premorbid period in the life of the affected individual. How far back does such a thrust imply? In the case of a child at risk for schizophrenia it is difficult to determine a specific time period, for one cannot specify precisely when an individual who will subsequently develop schizophrenia may be entirely free of early manifestations of the disorder. I recall a conference presentation by Mednick et al. (1971) in which the investigative team of one of the foremost risk studies in the world first presented their data on birth and perinatal complications in the biological offspring of schizophrenic mothers. One hypothesis set forth was that such complications potentiated the developmental lags noted in many of these vulnerable children at one year of age. In the commentaries that followed by Heston (1971) and Fish (1971), both asserted that an equally tenable hypothesis was that the developmental anomalies the investigators had reported were not necessarily expressions of a strictly environmental event acting on a genetically vulnerable infant but perhaps a manifestation of the schizophrenic genotype itself. Fish's comments illuminate the problem:

> I think of schizophrenia in the infant, of *early antecedents of schizophrenia* (italics added), or the vulnerable, heterozygous, possibly schizophrenic infants, as having a genetically determined central nervous system deviation which affects the regulation of all their growth patterns, including everything under control of the central nervous system—not only the autonomic nervous system but the entire developmental pattern. . . .
> It's possible that in some of these infants the active schizophrenic process, whatever it is, can start not simply at birth, but may begin before, and that the low birth weight may actually be one manifestation of existing schizophrenic illness, rather than being an external precipitating event (p. S119).

In a context of uncertainty as to how genetic structures are manifested in phenotypic behavior, the determination of what is viewed as premorbid becomes somewhat of a reflection of the beliefs, interests, and theoretical orientation of the risk researcher.

Where then does one begin? If one examines various ongoing programs of risk research one finds coverage of the entire age ranging from infancy through adolescence and early adulthood. Some investigators begin their research during the schizophrenic mother's pregnancy, and one investigator is even present during the birth of most offspring born to members of the maternal cohort. Still others begin their investigations during the early adolescence of the child at risk in the legitimate belief that by doing so their studies will provide insights into a period of development that immediately precedes one of the peak incidence rate periods for the emergence of overt schizophrenia. Others choose the middle years of childhood for their experimental scrutiny.

Elsewhere we have described the varying perspectives—genetic, psychological, sociological, and early deprivational patterns—that can serve as research models for the risk researcher (Garmezy and Streitman, 1974). Evidence in support of these models weighs differently for different types of risk. Delinquency and antisocial behavior seem to reflect the etiologic power of sociocultural and familial variables, but in the study of the most severe forms of adult psychopathology, particularly schizophrenia, the power of genetic factors is reflected in a number of classic studies that have appeared in recent years (e.g., Gottesman and Shields, 1972; Heston, 1966; Kety et al., 1968; Fischer, 1973). These studies provide a pragmatic basis for increasing the low base rate for the incidence of schizophrenia from approximately 1 percent in the general population to 10 to 12 percent in offspring born of a single schizophrenic parent. Truly high risk is present in those less frequent matings in which both parents have been schizophrenic. Offspring of such a union face a projected incidence figure that approximates 35 to 45 percent.

And yet case histories of the overwhelming majority of adult schizophrenic patients indicate that most (about 90 percent) have not had a schizophrenic parent. This very large population of individuals escape our selection networks, for we lack those genetic (or psychological) markers for schizophrenia that would then permit the preselection of children at risk. This difficulty is exacerbated by the inadequacy of alternative theoretical models that would complement or substitute for the genetic model. The nonspecificity of these models is such as to fail to provide the explicitness required to develop well-articulated criteria by which to select vulnerable children. It is this shortcoming that explains the current stereotypic preoccupation with the biological offspring of a parent who has been schizophrenic as *the* selection mode for defining risk for schizophrenia.

RESEARCH PROBLEMS IN STUDYING RISK FOR SCHIZOPHRENIA

The growth of risk studies in schizophrenia has made evident certain methodological problems that are very important yet do not negate the significance of the studies now under way. It is worth noting, however, that the risk researchers in schizophrenia, whose task is not an easy one to begin with, face some pressing methodological problems that add immeasurably to their burden:

1. In the case of risk for schizophrenia, there is in many instances a long waiting period between the observational and laboratory studies made in childhood and the emergence of disorder in adulthood. The risk period for schizophrenia extends to age 45, and more recently some have suggested that an extension to age 55 would be appropriate. Consider the dedication demanded of researchers who have to await the final determination of risk over a period that extends through decades. It is true, however, that a peak incidence for schizophrenia occurs in the late teens and early twenties and this ameliorates the problem somewhat. However, prognostically more favorable cases (which may reflect quite different antecedents) do occur in later adult life.

2. Hovering in the background is the ubiquitous problem of reliability of the parental diagnosis which often must be adjudged from inadequate case records marked by brief histories replete with contradictory or sparse information.

3. The ascertainment of offspring poses a problem too. Immigration, mobility downward (or upward) may result in irretrievable sample losses which are further accentuated by the placement of offspring of disturbed parents in foster homes or by their adoption by relatives or strangers.

4. The absence of any signs of disorder in many of the children at risk generates a pressing ethical question. Given the realities of informed consent, are the potential results to be obtained commen-

surate with the arousal of anxiety, guilt, and shame that may be generated in parents and children since identification and explanation of the purpose of one's project are required by committees on the use of human subjects in research?

5. An additional problem is generated by the small samples available to investigative teams, and this limitation inhibits broad generalizations. The need for a disturbed parent in selecting a biological offspring implies that one may be dealing with a fertile, more intact, certainly more cooperative parental cohort, and this too provides constraints in generalizing to the more fragmented world of many preschizophrenics who come out of far less competent backgrounds.

6. Data analysis based upon small Ns, the need to combine multiple subgroups that may vary in important ways, beyond a similarity in phenotypic behavior, such as the adaptive qualities of the nondisordered spouse, or the acuteness-chronicity dimension in the disordered spouse, poses problems of interpretation of results.

7. Finally, the absence of U.S. registries—psychiatric, adoption, and geographic—and marked restrictions in the contents and usage of those few that are available block the longitudinal pursuit of outcome in a markedly mobile United States.

Given these marked limitations, why the growing effort to assay studies of risk? As the discussant of a risk research symposium that constituted a portion of the program of the recently held Second Rochester International Conference on Schizophrenia, I attempted to answer a self-generated question (Garmezy, in press). What would be the consequences, I asked a panel of leading risk researchers, if 20 years from now the effort to map the lives of these vulnerable children revealed that we hadn't been able to predict the course of their disordered or nondisordered development at all? Would there have been any value gained from support of the multiple programs of risk research now under way?

I framed a reply through the mechanism of asking two other questions: (1) Did the research groups do a scholarly job of tracking the development of children born of schizophrenic parentage (or by the use of any alternative etiological model) through infancy, childhood, adolescence, and early maturity? (2) Had it proved possible to predict who in time became schizophrenic?

Clearly, if the answer to the first question was negative, the answer to the second question was most likely to be negative too. But if the answer to the first question proved to be an affirmative one, then even a negative response to question 2 would have made the venture into risk research worthwhile, for it would have provided for clinical psychiatry and developmental psychopathology the descriptive knowledge essential for understanding (1) the nature of predisposition to schizophrenia, and perhaps (2) the conditions required for its actualization, (3) the diversity of likely outcomes, and (4) the probable factors that influenced such diversity.

Such a contribution would be a first step toward the establishment of the developmental psychopathology envisioned by Piaget and others—an emergent developmental psychopathology parented by several disciplines and an offspring worthy to be welcomed to the ranks of emerging sciences.

INVULNERABLE CHILDREN IN THE CONTEXT OF RISK RESEARCH

I have suggested a diversity of probable outcomes for the child at risk for schizophrenia—although these outcomes are reflected in the genetic literature of schizophrenia, it remained for a great figure of European psychiatry to write an account of resistance to psychopathology with the clinical wisdom and compassion it requires.

Professor Manfred Bleuler is the great son of a great father. His lifework is the monumental achievement of creating a clinical-longitudinal research program in which he has ministered virtually as a family physician to 208 schizophrenic patients and their families. He has traced what has happened to these individuals over a span of two decades. Next year his volume (Bleuler, in press) on the results of his study will be published in English by Yale University Press with support funding provided by the Schizophrenia Research Program of the Scottish Rite. This five-year lag from the date of its original publication in German bests by 34 years the disconcerting delay in translation into English that followed upon the appearance in German of Eugen Bleuler's (1950) classic volume *Dementia Praecox or The Group of Schizophrenias.*

Professor Bleuler (1974) provided us with a preview in the *Schizophrenia Bulletin* of his observations on "The Offspring of Schizophrenics." In that chapter he noted that the occupational and marital lives of the 184 offspring of the 208 parents were often marked by a quality of competence and adaptation little anticipated on the basis of the stresses that they had endured as children. He writes:

> But despite the miserable childhoods described above, and despite their presumably "tainted" genes, most offspring of schizophrenics manage to lead normal productive lives. Indeed, after studying a number of family histories, one is left with the impression that pain and suffering can have a steeling—a hardening—effect on some children, rendering them capable of mastering life with all its obstacles, just to spite their inherent disadvantages. Perhaps it would be instructive for future investigators to keep as careful watch on the favorable development of the majority of these children as they do on the progressive deterioration of the sick minority.
>
> . . . One of the most lasting impressions brought home to me by the family studies of our subjects is the fact that even normal offspring who are successful in life can never fully free themselves from the pressures imposed by memories of their schizophrenic parents and their childhood. Once one knows them intimately, it is not rare to hear, as from the depths of their hearts, a long-drawn sigh, and something like: "When you've gone through that . . . you can never really be happy, you can never laugh as others do. You always have to be ashamed of yourself and take care not to break down yourself." Children of schizophrenics commonly feel that they are incompetent as partners in love or marriage, and could in no way assume the awesome responsibility of putting children of their own into the world. Many eventually overcome such inhibitions. But others never do; they plunge into their jobs and reject a normal family life.
>
> In short, the sufferings that children of schizophrenics endure can continue to affect their lives, even when they do not interfere with their health and professional advancement. Any hor-

rible experience remembered from childhood can continue to
hurt and to cast its shadow over life's happiness (p. 106).

Professor Bleuler has touched here on two points. The first is the
presence of resistance to psychopathology, or, perhaps stated more
dramatically, of invulnerability to disorder in some of these children;
the second point relates to the question of resistance—but at what
cost? So here, too, is the recognition of diversity of outcome even
among those who resist disorder, just as it has been observed among
those who capitulate to psychopathology. However, the fact that so
many children from severely disordered backgrounds can escape psychiatric breakdown should give us pause before we embark on simplistic etiological theorizing about "risk." The "steeling" effect noted
by Professor Bleuler demands equal time and equal study.

We have been guilty of almost a nonbenign neglect of these unusual children. Our neglect of the child who is adaptive under stress
reflects an orientation that Lois Murphy (1962) has long decried.
In *The Widening World of Childhood* she summed up our neglect
in this fashion:

> It is something of a paradox that a nation which has exulted in
> its scientific-technological achievements, should have developed
> in its studies of childhood so vast a "problem" literature: a litera-
> ture often expressing adjustment difficulties, social failure,
> blocked potentialities and defeat. . . . In applying clinical ways
> of thinking formulated out of experience with broken adults,
> we were slow to see how the language of adequacy to meet life's
> challenges could become the subject matter of psychological
> science. Thus there are thousands of studies of maladjustment for
> each one that deals directly with the ways of managing life's
> problems with personal strength and adequacy. The language
> of problems, difficulties, inadequacies, of antisocial or delinquent
> conduct, or of ambivalence and anxiety is familiar. We know
> that there are devices for correcting, bypassing, or overcoming
> threats, but for the most part these have not been directly
> studied (p. 2) .

One senses a Zeitgeist that will soon visibly reflect the shift from
the maladaptive to the adaptive, from high vulnerability to disorder

to apparent resistance to its manifestations, from emphasis on incompetence to one of maintaining and enhancing mastery. It would be ironic indeed if that shift and our growing awareness of how positive adaptations under crises are generated ultimately provided the tools for more effective intervention against behavioral disturbance in disordered children rather than the traditional therapeutic efforts that have engaged our attention for decades past.

REFERENCES

AINSWORTH, M. D. S. 1972. Attachment and dependency: A comparison. In J. L. Gewirtz (ed.), *Attachment and Dependency*, pp. 97-137. Washington, D.C.: Winston.

BELL, R. Q. 1968. A reinterpretation of the direction of effects in studies of socialization. *Psychol. Rev.*, 75:81-95.

BELL, R. Q. 1974. Contributions of human infants to caregiving and social interaction. In M. Lewis and L. A. Rosenblum (eds.), *The Effect of the Infant on Its Caregiver*, pp. 1-19. New York: Wiley.

BLEULER, E. 1950. *Dementia Praecox* or *The Group of Schizophrenias*. New York: International Universities Press.

BLEULER, M. 1974. The offspring of schizophrenics. *Schizophrenia Bull.* No. 8 (spring): 93-107.

BLEULER, M. *The Schizophrenic Mental Disorders in the Light of Long-Term Patient and Family Histories*. New Haven: Yale University Press (translated by Siegfried M. Clemens), in press.

BOWLBY, J. 1977. The making and breaking of affectional bonds. 1. Aetiology and psychopathology in the light of attachment theory. *Brit. J. Psychiatry*, 130:201-210.

FISCHER, M. 1973. Genetic and environmental factors in schizophrenia. *Acta Psychiatr. Scand.*, 238 (suppl.).

FISH, B. 1971. Genetic or traumatic developmental deviation? *Soc. Biol.* 18 (suppl.): S117-S119.

FREUD, S. 1920. The psychogenesis of a case of homosexuality in a woman. In S. Freud, *Collected Papers Vol. 2*, 1956, pp. 202-231. London: Hogarth Press.

GARMEZY, N. 1977. Vulnerable and invulnerable children. APA Master Lectures on Developmental Psychology. *Journal Supplement Abstraction Service*. Catalogue of Selected Documents in Psychology MS 1337. Washington, D.C.: American Psychological Association.

GARMEZY, N. Observations on high risk research and premorbid development in schizophrenia. In L. C. Wynne, R. Cromwell, and S. Matthysse (eds.), *Nature of Schizophrenia: New Findings and Future Strategies*. New York: Wiley, in press.

GARMEZY, N., and STREITMAN, S. 1974. Children at risk: The search for the antecedents of schizophrenia. Part I: Conceptual models and research methods. *Schizophrenia Bull.* No. 8:14-90.

GIL, D. G. 1970. *Violence Against Children: Physical Abuse in the United States.* Cambridge: Harvard University Press.

GOTTESMAN, I. I., and SHIELDS, J. 1972. *Schizophrenia & Genetics: A Twin Study Vantage-Point.* New York: Academic Press.

HESTON, L. L. 1966. Psychiatric disorders in foster home reared children of schizophrenic mothers. *Brit. J. Psychiatry*, 112:819-825.

HESTON, L. L. 1971. Schizophrenia—onset in infancy? *Soc. Biol.* 18 (suppl.):S114-S116.

JAYARATNE, S. 1977. Child abusers as parents and children: A review. *Social Work,* 22:5-9.

KETY, S. S., ROSENTHAL, D., SCHULSINGER, F., and WENDER, P. H. 1968. The types and prevalence of mental illness in the biological and adoptive families of adopted schizophrenics. *J. Psychiatr. Res.,* suppl. 1:345-362.

KLIEN, M., and STERN, L. 1971. Low birth weight and the battered child syndrome. *Am. J. Dis. Childhood,* 122:15-18.

LEWIS, M., and ROSENBLUM, L. A. (eds.). 1974. *The Effect of the Infant on Its Caregiver.* New York: Wiley.

MEDNICK, S., MURA, E., SCHULSINGER, F., and MEDNICK, B. 1971. Perinatal conditions and infant development in children with schizophrenic parents. *Soc. Biol.,* 18 (suppl.): S103-S113.

MEDNICK, S. A., and SCHULSINGER, F. 1973. Studies of children at high risk for schizophrenia. In S. R. Dean (ed.), *Schizophrenia: The First Ten Dean Award Lectures.* New York: MSS Information Corporation, pp. 247-293.

MURPHY, L. 1962. *The Widening World of Childhood.* New York: Basic Books.

PARKE, R. D., and COLLMER, C. W. 1975. Child abuse: An interdisciplinary analysis. In E. M. Hetherington, J. W. Hagen, R. Kron, and A. H. Stein (eds.), *Review of Child Development Research,* vol. 5, pp. 509-590. Chicago: University of Chicago Press.

PIAGET, J. 1975. Foreword. In E. J. Anthony (ed.), *Explorations in Child Psychiatry,* vii-ix. New York: Plenum.

SROUFE, L. A. The ontogenesis of emotion in infancy. In J. Osofsky (ed.), *Handbook of Infant Development.* New York: Wiley, in press.

SROUFE, L. A., and MITCHELL, P. Emotional development. In J. Osofsky (ed.), *Handbook of Infant Development.* New York: Wiley, in press.

SROUFE, L. A., and WATERS, E. *Attachment as an Organizational Construct.* Mimeographed. Minneapolis: University of Minnesota, in press.

STEELE, B. F., and POLLOCK, C. B. 1971. The battered child's parents. In A. S. Skolnick and J. H. Skolnick (eds.), *Families in Transition.* Boston: Little, Brown.

STEELE, B. F., and POLLOCK, C. B. 1974. A psychiatric study of parents who abuse infants and small children. In R. E. Helfer and C. H. Kempe (eds.), *The Battered Child,* 2nd Ed., pp. 89-133. Chicago: University of Chicago Press.

THOMAS, A., CHESS, S., and BIRCH, H. G. 1968. *Temperament and Behavior Disorders in Children.* New York: New York University Press.

5

Infant-Caretaker Interaction Research in an Inner City Community

MARGARET MORGAN LAWRENCE, M.D.

"If," write Condon and Sander (1974), "the infant from the beginning moves in precise shared rhythm with the organization of the speech structure of his culture, then he participates developmentally through complex, sociobiological entrainment processes in millions of repetitions of linguistic forms long before he will later use them in speaking and communicating. By the time he begins to speak he may have already laid down within himself the form and structure of the language system of his culture. This would encompass a multiplicity of interlocking aspects: rhythms and syntactic 'hierarchies,' suprasegmental features, paralinguistic nuances, not to mention body-motion styles and rhythms. . . . It thus suggests inquiry into the 'bond' between human beings as an expression of participation with shared organizational forms rather than as isolated entities, sending discrete messages."

"In the beginning was the Word." Through the "Word," infant-caretaker interactions are derived; ego functions are developed (Freud, 1936; de Hirsch, 1975); self-images and identities are achieved; feelings, pleasurable and unpleasurable, are confirmed, labeled and categorized (Stechler and Latz, 1966; Bennett, 1976). Observation of the infant's behavior may reveal true anxiety and an inner life of fantasy to match the action of key figures in the infant's outer world (Winnicott, 1975; Galenson, Miller and Roiphe, 1976). Through the Word, object relationships are established.

71

Winnicott (1971) posits the development of an intermediary zone between infant and object, "between inner and outer reality" (p. 4), in which the inner life of both parties participates. It is in this intermediary zone between the inner and outer life of both that the interaction occurs, pleasurable or unpleasurable. This is "play" (M. M. Lawrence, 1971, pp. 30-32). It has the character of "dreamwork" shared by patient and analyst. "Psychotherapy takes place in the overlap of two areas of playing, that of the patient and that of the therapist" (Winnicott, 1971, p. 38). When a young child, even an infant, has perceived and experienced trauma, such as separation and the physical trauma of child battery, with the feelings of anger, sadness, and anxiety that accompany the trauma, it is possible for infant and caretaker or infant and therapist to apperceive, to review the trauma in a shared dramatic act. This act is a play whose accompaniment of words, movement, and high feeling-tone help resolve feelings related to the trauma. Winnicott (1975) describes the relief of asthma symptoms in a seven-month-old during the observation of the infant in a set situation. In my own experience I have referred to sharing of a known traumatic experience and its attached feelings with a young child or infant as "catharsis for feelings." This is always done in the context of readily available support and awareness of adequate ego strength in the infant or child.

Through the Word, the bodily proximity that it brings, the experience and change in movement, and the feeling-tones of the infant bearer, are mediated personal love and concern, the supports of family, extended family and community, the ills of poverty, the hopes of the civil-rights era, the demands of black pride and power—indeed the psychodynamics, the histories, and culture of generations past projected into the faith and hopes of caretakers for the future. It is here, therefore, in this humanizing intervention, that prevention of developmental ills, treatment with respect to deficits of nature and nurturing, and identification of ego strength are possible.

The news of my granddaughter's birth came as my husband and I sat in the airport in Nairobi, Kenya, on February 2, 1973. We were en route to Dar es Salaam. The cable read, "It's a girl." Then followed her name, which we later learned was of South African origin. Her parents translated it for us. Our granddaughter's name means "Lovely Hope." It was partially at our son's and daughter-in-law's insistence that we had made this trek to the "mother land," West and East Africa. They had journeyed there four times, and on the last trip had engaged in serious study. Visiting secondary schools, they had inquired in what way the traditions and heritage of the families represented in each school had proved helpful in building a modern institution.

Ten years before our trip to Africa, in 1963, I had returned to Harlem Hospital Center for the first time since my residency there in pediatrics. The Department of Psychiatry had recently become affiliated with that at Columbia University. We organized a Developmental Psychiatry Service for children under five and their families within the Division of Child Psychiatry. During the last five years of the ten between my homecoming at Harlem and my trip to Africa, names like the one my granddaughter bears became commonplace among the black poor. These names spoke of black pride and black power. Small boys who were markedly aggressive and verbal, as well as those who because of minimal brain dysfunction were nonverbal, bore such names as Hasson (warrior) and Taikuma (courageous). Some mothers and fathers of these boys, well identified with concerns for black pride, were lifting themselves educationally by their bootstraps. Other mothers at first look appeared shy and retiring. A deeper look revealed their assertive and aggressive drives. It was as if their aggressive "little men" spoke for them. Meanwhile, these same mothers presented complaints about their sons' misbehavior. Fathers also delegated their power to their sons in the same manner. Girls were given African names that referred to feminine beauty and grace.

In my own upbringing in Mississippi I had been well aware of the relationship between the names given infants at birth and parents' hopes and expectations of these children. Through children's names adults communicated the images they held of them, such as Precious Jewel. A brief study in 1972-73 of the "identifiable strengths of black preschool children and their families which may survive their special risks" took me again to Mississippi and Georgia. One four-year-old in a Rankin County, Mississippi, daycare center volunteered, "My mother calls me Princess." Her father had hauled the cement blocks for the building of his children's daycare center. He participated in the rebuilding of churches in the area bombed out not many years ago. Parents and communities found their own worth in building for their children and themselves. These same people marched with their children to Washington in 1967.

Sandy Hopper also attended the Rankin County Community Day Care Center. He lived deep in the pines some distance from the gravel road. Sandy's house resembled a small box standing on stilts. He, his mother, and his two-year-old sister lived there. No father was visible. I told Sandy's mother that Mrs. Smith, the director, had picked Sandy because he is a strong boy. I added, "He must have a strong family."

Ms. Hopper told me Sandy had been named for her grandfather who had helped to organize the Charlie Harrison Bowler High School, the first black high school in Newton County. "He was *mean,*" Ms. Hopper said. "I'm mean like him, and Sandy too." I interrupted, "You say *mean,* maybe 'tough,' 'strong' like Sandy." "Yes," she agreed. The director had said, "Sandy has all the energy you can find anywhere. He is 'hard-headed,' too."

I engaged Sandy in a family play using family dolls and furniture on the floor of the director's office. The play was audiotaped and I also took notes. I summarized: Sandy was able to show dramatic action in his play, but was largely silent throughout the first half. He became more and more expressive during the second half of his play, permitting himself to play with the small plastic dinosaurs and calling them "mice." Significant to Sandy's ego strength were both his "mean" great grandfather, for whom he was named, although he had never seen him, and his road-construction worker grandfather who, in spite of being away "on the road" for months at a time, provided Sandy and his family with considerable economic and emotional support. Sandy's mother had been for five years an attendant in the neighboring state mental hospital; her sister and a paid baby sitter had helped her with the care of the children.

Sandy was not the "son of a woman," the epithet used in anger among boys at Mama Gina Kenyatta's Childrens' Home in Nairobi, Kenya. A "son of a woman" is a boy whose father is unknown, that is, a boy who is felt to be virtually without male identity. So untenable is the position of such a boy in the home that the staff includes both a headmaster and a female director. Adult male "friends" or "pals" make regular visits to boys who have no known male relatives. In Nigeria, a sociologist at the University of Ife confirmed the importance of the fathering role. A then-current newspaper reported that three different men were suing to establish their paternity of one infant.

Fathers of young children can be found in the Harlem Hospital community if one conscientiously looks outside of the hospital for them, if they appear unwilling to come in. A black Muslim father brought his bright but nonverbal three-year-old son to us for evaluation. His son's mother, his girl friend, had left him to go into the army and to marry another. This father responsibly met the requirements of the clinic for the evaluation of his son. In the boy's general care the father had the support of both of the boy's grandmothers.

Schecter (1974) writes, "Parental hopes for their offspring are universal and have been expressed in the form of the messianic ideal; this theme runs through various religious, mythological, and artistic motifs throughout history" (p. 268). Arlow states, "identifications with heroes or heroines of the classic or central myths point the way to the establishment of ego ideals and superego structures in consonance with the moral traditions of the society" (1964, p. 13). Miss Pittman, a black woman born in slavery in the film, *The Autobiography of Miss Jane Pittman,* cradled a black manchild on her lap. "She asked of herself, the small group that surrounded her, and the child himself, 'Is this . . . Are you the one?' " (M. M. Lawrence, 1976)

I have elsewhere described (Lawrence, 1975) young families, chiefly poor and black, in the Harlem Hospital community. "Strength abounds in these families, and it, too, is a reflection, to some extent, of the survival of an inherited strength by all the avenues open to inheritance: nature, nurture and culture" (p. 131). The history, culture, and myths of a people, "the stuff of life itself," can make available to those who share it their own ego strengths, even persons "at high risk." It is for us who study and serve among such persons to help them to recognize these riches. Openness to their history, culture, and myths helps us to turn from a dehumanizing approach born of our own despair to a more humanizing attitude toward the poor with whom we work and study. The first question asked of a parent in a diagnostic family evaluation initiated to study the developmental problems of a preschool child may be "Where did you come from?" And as we meet families, we remain expectant of finding the family's men. Recently 10 of the 18 families represented in our therapeutic nursery gave a day-long dinner sale which they aptly named "We Sell Soul." Parents and staff provided the food. Four fathers worked all day delivering dinners and cooking in the nursery kitchen with the mothers. Net receipts were $375.

Of our 20 two- to five-year-old children, almost all of whom have mild organic problems that may be called minimal brain dysfunction, only two exhibit autistic features that lead us to make the diagnosis of borderline autism. Ornitz and Ritvo (1976) deny that deficient human stimulation, for example, maternal deprivation, may cause autism. "While environmental deprivation has been shown to induce serious developmental disturbances, it does not produce the syndrome of autism," they write (p. 613). Because of our assumption that interferences in communication between infant or child and caretaker as a result of constitutional inadequacy or minimal brain dysfunction, closely related to maternal and social deprivation, may lead to autism, we continue to inquire into the infrequency of this disorder in our population.

In a pediatric ward of the Muhumbili Hospital in Dar es Salaam in 1973, mothers and babies were receiving medical treatment for malnutrition. Mothers also learned to cook nourishing foods grown in the region in a small round "palaver" outside the ward. They had traveled with the babies for many miles to bring them to the hospital. Thin and gaunt, with empty, sagging breasts, these women walked about the ward, carrying their babies either on their backs or at their breasts. The babies looked cadaverous, with large bellies, their thin skin parched. None cried. I asked the Nigerian pediatrician there, "How much autism do you see in Tanzania or Nigeria?" "None," was the crisp reply. "And why?" I asked. Patiently, he answered, "They carry their babies on their backs until they are two."

In Mississippi I learned to soothe an infant on my lap with a nontiring, gentle, rhythmic lifting of my knees, or to sway back and forth with an infant in arms as I sat in a straight chair. Mothers, grandmothers, and neighbors felt free to "pacify" a baby, to feed him bits of food, to sing "sorrow songs" to him. Posture, bodies, movement were a part of the baby's environment.

Not only were positive feelings shared with infants in play, but the adult's negative emotions were also part of the infants' lives. Babies at the breast and knee babies too were touched and held by the bereaved mother as neighbors "paid respects." The deceased in those days was "laid out" in the same room.

C. R. Lawrence writes (personal communication, 1976), "All interaction among human beings takes place within cultural and historical contexts. Ways of thinking and behaving are transmitted from one generation to the next in the process of social interaction. Norms of conduct, i.e., expected behavior under particular circumstances, vary by societies and by groups within societies; and this is as true of infant-caretaker interaction as it is of other human behavior.

"The families seen and treated at Harlem Hospital Center are part of the general western/North American/United States culture and, therefore, share general American norms regarding desirable and undesirable behavior, the importance of success or failure, and a hierarchy of values regarding goods and services. They are also part of a subculture which is influenced by the historical origins of these families in the Southern United States and the Caribbean. And the varying degrees of racial discrimination, oppression, and self-understandings of these regions are also part of this social inheritance.

"The present objective socioeconomic situations of the families are also part of this cultural-historical context. As low-income members of America's non-white urban population, for example, a high proportion of the infants will come from one-parent, female-headed households. Their families are generally poor.

"Much has been written in recent years about the 'culture of poverty' with its self-perpetuating cycle of poverty-dependency (Moynihan, 1965; Rainwater, 1970; Schulz, 1969). The culture of poverty perspective has tended to see the poor as an almost separate culture, often ignoring the large body of common cultural assumptions which they share with the rest of the population and generally oblivious to the presence of ego strength among even the very poor. There are frequently implications that all of the poor—particularly the black poor—are part of this 'culture of poverty.' Fortunately, this view is beginning to be corrected (Lewis, 1967; C. R. Lawrence, 1971; Hill, 1972; M. M. Lawrence, 1975; Valentine, 1968)."

Bernard (1971) wrote, ". . . to deny in effect that unconscious conflicts, as well as external stresses, contribute to symptoms, dysfunctions, and distress on the part of those who are underprivileged is to inflict still another subtle form of discrimination upon them; it is as though one were saying that, in their case, the fundamentals of psychiatry, as to psychic structure and function (including malfunction), do not apply" (p. 76).

"The Harlem community," I wrote in 1975, "requires our best understanding of familial and developmental dynamics, unconscious conflicts and dated emotions, the creation of self-images and the roles and limitations of drives, ideals, and goals. This knowledge is needed in the infant day-care center as well as the carpeted nursery" (p. 55).

Five-year-old Leon's borderline autism can be traced to his mother's feelings of rejection in her own family of orientation. She felt "left out" by both parents, growing up with six siblings "down South." She married a Vietnam veteran whose anger at returning to this country's social scene precipitated a brawl with friends and the loss of his job. During Leon's mother's pregnancy with him, her beloved next older sister died. "This sister," Mrs. Johnson said, "was the only one who cared about me." Later the same sister's baby died. Leon was born between his aunt's and his cousin's death. Mrs. Johnson spent Leon's first year holding him in her arms and watching television. In an interview with the Johnson family of three, Leon wrapped a doll in a blanket and handed it to his father. Both parents have slowly proved their ability to profit by the insight gained concerning their own psychodynamics. Slowly, too, their ego strengths have become available to their family.

Dr. Stephen Bennett initiated an Infant Psychiatry Unit in Harlem's Developmental Psychiatry Service two years ago. Our first task was to consult with various pediatric staff members concerning infants on the pediatric wards, chiefly "boarder babies." These babies sometimes remain in the hospital nursery up to four months of age. They are chiefly infants of drug-addicted mothers. Their delay in leaving the hospital is often caused by the lack of a decision concerning foster care placement on the part of the Bureau of Child Welfare. Some of these babies, small and drug-influenced at birth, spend their early weeks in an incubator for premature infants. A month later, as they arrive at the "boarder baby" nursery, they may be well-nourished, but unresponsive.

For the past year the Infant Psychiatry Unit has conducted monthly seminars that are interdisciplinary and interdepartmental. All departments and disciplines share a concern for improved infant-caretaker interaction in the maladaptive infant-caretaker pair. Maladaptive mothers may be addicted, psychotic, or in their early adolescence. Infants may show aberrant development.

We are initiating an early intervention study whose main focus is to observe and record the emergence of early affective behavior in high-risk infants in response to their caretakers and in the context of familial and extended family life, their history and culture, and with full attention to the psychodynamics of the chief caretakers.

Our study combines the microanalysis, or the method of "frame by frame film analysis" of Stern (1976) in the study of infant-caretaker interaction (p. 113), with the study of familial psychodynamics, history and culture, as described. What are the effects of deficits existing in mother, infant, family, and community, including deficits in nurturing over several generations, on infant-caretaker interaction? Are we able to identify ego strengths and show their role in infant-caretaker interaction?

Bennett (1976) describes the behavior of three black infants in the early weeks of life who are in the charge of child-caring persons in a "boarder baby" nursery. He graphically points to the marked influence of caretaker attitudes and expectations on the three babies. "The basic personality given Smitty, as he was quickly nicknamed, was friendliness and good nature. Early the most frequent comment was, 'He's a smart baby' " (p. 82). This author immediately recognizes that the caretakers are black. Since and perhaps during slavery, since the same attitude exists today among the village committee of the daycare center in Kiambu province in Kenya, no Afro-American has questioned the need for a "headstart" for the child he or she bounces gently on a knee. Every movement of the cradling body sings: "You are the one."

REFERENCES

ARLOW, J. A. 1964. The Madonna's conception through the eyes. *The Psychoanalytic Study of Society*, 3:13-25.

BENNETT, S. L. 1976. Infant-caretaker interactions. In E. N. Rexford, L. W. Sander, and T. Shapiro (eds.), *Infant Psychiatry*, pp. 79-98. New Haven: Yale University Press.

BERNARD, V. W. 1971. Composite remedies for psycho-social problems in psychiatric care of the underprivileged. In G. Belasso (ed.), *International Psychiatry Clinics*, pp. 61-85. Boston: Little, Brown.

CONDON, W. S., and SANDER, L. W. 1974. Synchrony demonstrated between movements of the neonate and adult speech. *Child Dev.*, 45:456-462.

DE HIRSCH, K. 1975. Language deficits in children. *Psychoanal. Study Child*, 30:95-123.

FREUD, A. 1936. *Ego and the Mechanism of Defense*. Tr. by L. Peller, 1946. New York: International Universities Press.

GALENSON, E., MILLER, R., and ROIPHE, H. 1976. The choice of symbols. *J. Am. Acad. Child Psychiatry*, 15:83-96.

HILL, R. 1972. *The Strength of Black Families*. New York: Emerson and Hall.

LAWRENCE, C. R. 1971. Color, class and culture: A minority view. In D. L. Grummon and A. M. Barclay (eds.), *Sexuality: A Search for Perspective*, pp. 109-125. New York: Van Nostrand Reinhold.

LAWRENCE, M. M. 1971. *Mental Health Team in the Schools*. New York: Behavioral Publications.

LAWRENCE, M. M. 1975. *Young Inner City Families: Development of Ego Strength Under Stress*. New York: Behavioral Publications.

LAWRENCE, M. M. 1976. The appraisal of ego strength in evaluation, treatment and consultation "Is This the One?" *J. Am. Acad. Child Psychiatry*, 15:1-14.

LEWIS, H. G. 1967. The family: Resources for change. In L. Rainwater and W. L. Yancey (eds.), *The Moynihan Report and the Politics of Controversy*. Cambridge: Massachusetts Institute of Technology Press.

MOYNIHAN, D. P. 1965. *The Negro Family: The Case for National Action*. Washington: U.S. Department of Labor, Office of Planning and Research.

ORNITZ, E. M., and RITVO, E. R. 1976. The syndrome of autism: A critical review. *Am. J. Psychiatry*, 133:609-621.

RAINWATER, L. 1970. *Behind Ghetto Walls*. Chicago: Aldine.

SCHECTER, D. E. 1974. Infant Development. In S. Arieti (ed.), *The American Handbook of Psychiatry*, 2nd Ed., 1:264-283.

SCHULZ, D. A. 1969. *Coming Up Black*. Englewood Cliffs, N.J.: Prentice-Hall.

STECHLER, G. S., and LATZ, E. 1966. Some observations on attention and arousal in the human infant. *J. Am. Acad. Child Psychiatry*, 5:517-525.

STERN, D. N. 1976. A microanalysis of mother-infant interaction. In E. N. Rexford, L. W. Sander, and T. Shapiro (eds.), *Infant Psychiatry*, pp. 113-126. New Haven: Yale University Press.

VALENTINE, C. 1968. *Culture of Poverty*. Chicago: University of Chicago Press.

WINNICOTT, D. W. 1971. *Playing and Reality*. New York: Basic Books.

WINNICOTT, D. W. 1975. *Through Pediatrics to Psychoanalysis*. New York: Basic Books.

Part III
THERAPEUTIC INTERVENTION RESEARCH

6

Reassessment of Eclecticism in Child Psychiatric Treatment

SAUL I. HARRISON, M.D.

More than twenty-five years ago, when I began serious study and work in psychiatry and child psychiatry, I learned very quickly that there was a type of psychiatrist I should not strive to be: an *eclectic* one. The connotation within the field was that eclectic psychiatrists were superficial and, because of their inadequate knowledge about too wide a range, ineffective. The dictionary definition of the word emphasizing "selectivity" was thoroughly overshadowed by this pejorative aura. The desirable alternative presented to me and to everyone else I knew at that time was to become a psychodynamically oriented child psychiatrist. Essentially, it was a simple choice between "good" and "bad"!

To indicate that this was not an idiosyncratic sentiment stemming from my admittedly limited perspective, it may be noted that in 1960 when the Committee on Medical Education of the Group for Advancement of Psychiatry (GAP) (1962) solicited the opinions of 91 heads of psychiatry departments regarding their psychological frame of reference, all 91 indicated that it was psychodynamic. More recently, in the course of reviewing and analyzing the National Insti-

This essay was conceived and written while the author was editing the Therapeutic Intervention Section of the *Basic Handbook of Child Psychiatry* (Basic Books, in press). In consequence, there is overlap of both thought and language between the introductory overview to that section and this essay. The author acknowledges with appreciation the helpful advice offered by Drs. Charles Davenport, Harvey Falit, Thomas Horner, Joseph Noshpitz, Elva Posnanski, Andrew Watson, and David Zinn.

tute of Mental Health's quarter-century of active leadership in the field, NIMH's Research Task Force (1975) sketched a picture of the late 1940s and early 1950s in which psychoanalysis and its derivative psychodynamic psychotherapies were the most developed forms of psychosocial treatment, behavior modification had not yet emerged from the laboratory, and the primary somatic treatments included electroconvulsive therapy, insulin coma, and lobotomy. Twenty-five years ago, effective treatments were available for central nervous system syphilis and the psychosis accompanying pellagra; for the most part, however, the few psychopharmacological agents at hand then were typically employed to manage rather than to treat patients.

Since then, there has been a phenomenal burgeoning of available therapeutic modalities. Evidence of what appears to be an expansion of exponential proportions comes from sources as disparate as the popular media, professional journals, and verbal reports. In the mid-1960s Harrison and Carek (1966) listed 70 psychotherapies that claimed distinctiveness (often with minimal justification), whereas less than a decade later NIMH's Research Task Force (1975) tallied more than 130 therapies. Without distinguishing between psychiatric treatment for adults and children, the task force characterized it as "vastly changed" and "revolutionized."

Thus it was no great challenge 25 years ago to be a versatile, all-encompassing psychiatric practitioner. Today such an accomplishment is barely within the reach of even the most knowledgeable and gifted child psychiatrist. It would not be a rash prediction to assert that soon it will be utterly impossible for any one person to be a Renaissance practitioner of child psychiatry capable of mastering all reasonable therapeutic interventions. Our question today is how the child psychiatric clinician should adapt to that change and contribute to its enhancement and refinement.

Proposals of methods to cope with the constantly expanding diversity of available therapeutic interventions readily polarize into two prevailing suggestions. One asserts that comparison of the outcome of different treatments (with the exception of pharmacological therapy) reveals insufficient differences on which to base discriminative specific therapeutic prescriptions. Thus far, objective studies make it appear that whatever the convinced clinician does with enthusiasm proves to be equally effective (e.g., Frank, 1961). Therefore, clinicians should employ those treatments they believe they do well and in which they have confidence. Indeed, this answer to our central question constitutes a fair representation of the thrust of most child psychiatric practice in the past.

The other answer occupies an opposite pole and will constitute the thesis of this essay. Before asserting it, I want to emphasize that I do not intend to diminish the significance of the therapist's competence, enthusiasm, and expectations. Nor do I intend to minimize child psychiatry's dire need for more research and its interrelation with clinical application. I do advocate that consideration be given also to the likelihood that the outcome of different therapies, as indicated by comparative studies which enabled Luborsky, Singer, and Luborsky (1975) to conclude, like the dodo bird of Alice in Wonderland, that "everybody has won and all must have prizes," may be attributed to factors other than similarities inherent in all of the treatments, such as the helping relationship with the therapist. Most significantly, the similarity of outcome might arise from the fact that there has been very little that is specific and discriminating in the prescription of different treatments for different disturbances. It seems clear that the choice of treatment stems far more often from the therapeutic-professional system's institutional or personal preferences than from an assessment of the recipients' individual differences.

The critical tenor of this commentary does not indicate that this essay will advocate that child psychiatrists try to apply treatments for which they are ill prepared and not qualified. Its intent is rather to urge child psychiatrists to be open and ready to consider a wide variety of treatments in the course of clinical assessments. In this way we may be more likely to match the individual child and/or family and their disturbance with the most appropriate specific therapeutic intervention. This may mean that the evaluating child psychiatrist is not qualified to implement the recommended treatment or combination of treatments himself and will have to arrange for some other clinician (s) to administer it.

Expounding the advantage of specificity of therapeutic differentiation requires a sober reassessment and perhaps a reorientation of attitudes toward eclecticism. This should entail more than modifying "eclectic" with qualifiers like "in the best sense of the word." Nor should such a reconsideration be misconstrued as asserting that child psychiatrists become eclectic in every—or in fact, in any—sense of the word. What is advocated is modification of automatic negative reactions to those aspects of eclecticism that emphasize pluralism and selectivity. Further, nothing that follows should be interpreted as advocating that child psychiatrists function without a preferred theory. Indeed, such a framework is required to organize the inevitably massive data of clinical observation. Along with our need for a theoretical framework, it is essential that we be vigilant that the theory not distort what we observe clinically nor influence the recommended intervention.

NIMH's Research Task Force observed that the addition of new treatments has not been accompanied by discarding old ones. Juxtaposing this observation with the paucity of clinically meaningful, methodologically sound, rigorously executed investigations that publicly document the value of most of the treatments highlights the wide gap separating these findings from the results reported by committed clinicians who are convinced of the treatment's value. At this juncture, it is helpful to recall that there are other conditions in which pluralistic treatments are the rule. These range from the difficult-to-treat cancers to the much more easily remedied styes in the eye for which one can nevertheless employ various combinations of hot compresses, local pressure, local antibiotics, sun glasses to prevent squinting, prescriptions for subclinical stigmatism, surgery, etc.

HISTORICAL PERSPECTIVE

Historically, the existence of a multiplicity of treatments for a given condition tends to have a high correlation with limited effectiveness for all of them. In addition, whenever a truly definitive child psychiatric treatment appeared in the past, such as the dietary measures for phenylketonuria, this resulted in responsibility for administration of the treatment being assigned to pediatrics. This situation also arises in adult psychiatry and internal medicine, as exemplified by pellagra and central nervous system syphilis. Perhaps this is consistent with the fact that, in both pediatrics and internal medicine, the major intellectual challenge is posed by diagnostic work; indeed, this tends to outweigh by far the relative simplicity of administering treatment. The opposite condition has prevailed in psychodynamic psychiatric work; treatment tends to be the most intellectually demanding clinical activity as well as potentially the most rewarding and most frustrating. The development of more specific child psychiatric treatments, however, increases the importance of the subtleties of diagnostic assessment. In adult psychiatry this has been illustrated most vividly by the American tendency, before the development of phenothiazines, monoamine oxidase inhibitors, tricyclics and lithium, not to distinguish carefully between schizophrenic and manic-depressive psychoses and to endeavor to substitute the all encompassing concept of schizo-affective reactions. One might risk a prediction that, in the future, diagnostic efforts might be expanded to include quantitative determination of the responsible neurotransmitter, its site of action, etc. While in this futuristic mode, it should be noted that although it is conceivable today that physiochemical genetics or therapy might some day ameliorate or even eliminate mental illness, it seems unlikely that enzymes or other functional macromolecules could by themselves undo the effects of pathogenic experiences without a simultaneous process of unlearning and relearning akin to some of the psychosocial therapies. As Seymour Kety (1960) speculated, "There may someday be a biochemistry or a biophysics of memory—but not of memories."

These comments highlight that the "revolutionizing" referred to in the NIMH report pertains more to psychiatric treatment of adult patients than to that of children. Consequently, it is worth emphasizing that innovative therapeutic efforts with children have frequently served as the cutting edge of conceptual and therapeutic advances. The early history of the development of many psychiatric treatment modalities is marked by accounts of treatment of children.

This statement impresses many as both surprising and inaccurate, because in the subsequent development of the treatment modality, child psychiatric work frequently has not sustained its leadership role. With the passage of time, psychiatric work with adults has tended to assume the lead, obscuring the earlier seminal child psychiatric contribution.

For instance, currently the treatment of major mental disorders in adults with psychotropic drugs appears far ahead of psychopharmacological treatment of children's disorders. It is thus all too easy to forget that pioneering work in clinical psychopharmacology, and the one that has withstood the test of time longest, is Charles Bradley's (1937) introduction of amphetamines for the treatment of disturbed children.

Similarly, modern community psychiatric activities, despite being faulted today for deemphasizing children's clinical needs (Cohen et al., 1975) have significant conceptual and pragmatic roots in the child guidance clinic movement of the 1920s. At its inception, child guidance emphasized its preventive role, its community consultative responsibility, and outreach activities. In particular, it was the main site for the development of the mental health team approach.

Another outgrowth of these early child psychiatric tactics is the active involvement of the identified patient's family in the diagnostic and therapeutic work. Eventually, this led to the development of family therapy, again pioneered in the context of work with disturbed children, as exemplified by Ackerman's (1958) seminal contributions. Again too, as McDermott and Char (1974) remind us, the burgeoning family therapy field and its evolving systems orientation are often perceived today as neglecting the young children in the family.

Another example of the vanguard role played by the treatment of children is the recent resurgence of behaviorism and its fruitful application to treatment techniques. This is rooted clinically in the demonstration by Mary Cover Jones (1924) more than 50 years ago that an infant who had been conditioned to fear furry objects (similar to the earlier demonstration by Watson and Raynor [1920] of the development of a phobia in the infant Albert) could be relieved of the fear by social imitation and direct reconditioning. The Mowrers' (1938) pad technique of treating enuresis was one of the earliest and most enduring behavioral therapeutic techniques and technological devices.

Bettelheim and Sylvester's (1948, 1949) development of the concept of a therapeutic milieu and the practice of milieu therapy represents a rare instance in which the fruitful adaptation of a method to adult psychiatry (e.g., Jones, 1953) has not overshadowed the work with children.

There are two notable exceptions to the generalization about work with children serving as the leading edge of innovative therapeutic developments. They are the nonpharmacological biological treatments and the development of psychoanalysis (and its historical antecedent and companion, hypnosis). Freud's pioneering work was with adults and older adolescents. To be sure, the seminal case report in 1909 of little Hans is responsible for ushering in the modern era of child psychotherapy; nonetheless, that was really an example of filial therapy. Freud asserted without equivocation that he was the adviser, that the young patient's father was the psychotherapist, and that the intimacy of the parent-child relationship was a vital prerequisite for the therapist (Freud, 1909). The first reported attempt of direct psychoanalytic treatment of a child without the use of a parental intermediary was published in 1913. In that case history, Ferenczi (1913) indicated that the psychoanalytic method, as then used with adults, could not be employed with his five-year-old patient, who rapidly became bored and wanted to return to his play. Eight years after Ferenczi's abortive effort, Hug-Hellmuth (1921) reported the use of play in the treatment of emotionally disturbed children. The role of play in the development of modern child psychotherapy has been compared to the historical significance of hypnosis in facilitating the understanding of unconscious mental functioning in adult psychiatry. Child psychoanalysis has subsequently been elaborated in different directions under the leadership of Anna Freud and Melanie Klein.

Simultaneously, in the United States in the 1920s, under the aegis of the Commonwealth Fund and Clifford Beer's National Committee for Mental Hygiene, child guidance clinics sprang up everywhere. Their form was modeled after William Healey's child psychiatric work at the juvenile court in Chicago and subsequently at the Judge Baker Clinic in Boston. Enriched by psychoanalytic developments in Europe, the child guidance clinic movement contributed to enlarging and expanding the scope of psychotherapeutic efforts with children.

CLINICAL SPECIFICITY

Although child psychiatric nosology has been refined and elaborated over the years, it nevertheless remains unfortunately limited primarily to classifying clinical description. At best, it has minimal explanatory value regarding etiology or indications for treatment (GAP, 1966; Rutter et al., 1969). In consequence, it is relatively simple to assign an appropriate diagnostic label. As the GAP report (1966) noted, at our current level of knowledge it is impossible to devise an ideal, universally useful diagnostic classificatory system encompassing syntheses of the clinical descriptive observations with psychodynamic, psychosocial, psychobiological, developmental, etiologic, prognostic, and therapeutic considerations. In spite of this, child psychiatrists need to match the individual child and his disturbance to specific therapeutic interventions. Irrespective of the orientation, training, and ideology of the clinician, this is the intended outcome of diagnostic assessment.

Compounding these limitations of the value of diagnostic labels is the imprecision concerning just what it is about a given therapeutic intervention that is curative. This uncertainty is illustrated vividly when one reviews the history of different therapeutic methods and observes how numerous factors have alternately been lauded as essential for therapeutic effectiveness and then damned as useless. Early in this century and preceding the ascendancy of psychoanalysis, the most prominent factors within the psychological framework were suggestions, persuasive exhortation, and reassurance. Then, when psychoanalysis first appeared, beneficial results were thought to be a consequence of rediscovering a lost memory along with the abreactive release of dammed-up emotions. Later developments in psychoanalytic thinking saw the emphasis shift to modification of superego standards, identification with the therapist, resolution of transference, increasing emotional discipline in the working-through process, insight, the analysis of defenses, and expansion of ego functioning. Concurrently, there has been a similar waxing and waning of attention to learning-behavioral, social, and biological factors.

Although they are derived from different conceptual frameworks and expressed in markedly different languages, some of the aforementioned factors show considerable overlap. It is inconceivable that all therapeutic progress with all patients can ever be the product of a unitary therapeutic factor; by the same token, it is highly unlikely that a single therapeutic element ever operates in isolation. Invariably, there are other influences simultaneously at work. For instance, the therapeutic relationship itself inevitably gives rise to corrective emotional experiences. These need not have been explicitly designed by the therapist; indeed, they may be an accidental by-product of the clinician's empathic posture. Nonetheless, the therapeutic relationship invariably exerts some influence.

Unfortunately, a tradition has grown up of mutual exclusivity of different therapeutic modalities. This has lead to pseudopolarities between therapeutic approaches. Child psychiatric educational programs are all too frequently unidimensional. In a field burdened by ambiguity, the very process of learning tends to evoke discomfort and uncertainty. This in turn encourages student clinicians to attempt to cope with their distress by jumping aboard what Halleck and Woods (1962) designated a "bandwagon" therapy, a process that can readily turn into what Klagsbrun (1967) labeled a "Garden of Eden" therapy. For the student, there is now only one truth. Such an allegiance reduces the student clinician's anxiety, is self-reinforcing, and often enjoys institutional support. This search for an illusory certainty risks compromising the clinician's empathic sensitivity; as Adams (1974) noted, it can result in forms of egocentrism on the part of both the clinician and the young patient which are remarkable for their similarity. This analogy is based on Piaget's (1932) observation that as a consequence of the nature of the relationship between child and adult, the child's thinking tends to be isolated. This places the child apart; while the child believes he/she is sharing the point of view of the world at large, he/she actually remains shut off and isolated in his/her own viewpoint.

VARIETIES OF THERAPEUTIC MODALITIES

To the extent that a clinician remains committed to a specific value set, he is likely to combine only certain therapeutic modes while excluding others from among the wide array of choices encompassing the psychodynamically oriented exploratory psychotherapies, supportive psychotherapies, brief time-limited psychotherapies, family therapy, filial therapy, parent counseling and/or therapy, the variety of behavior therapies, the group therapies, a range of pharmacotherapeutic agents, milieu therapy, a multitude of psychoeducational approaches, special symptom-focused remediation such as tutoring or speech therapy, hypnotherapy, biofeedback, and on and on. It cannot be stressed too frequently that the use of these approaches, singly or in combination, should stem less from the clinician's preferences than from the assessment of the patient.

Lists of therapeutic modalities like the foregoing incomplete one inevitably reflect an isolating tendency comparable in some respects to what Piaget described for children. On one hand, the field of child psychiatric treatment may easily be perceived as a state of undisciplined chaos; on the other, however, any effort to bring order to it risks creating an oversimplified form of tunnel vision. This would not serve the clinician, who in practice must embrace a shifting pluralism which encompasses sociology, various types of psychology, genetics, biochemistry, physiology, etc. Since these disciplines all employ different concepts and language, this demands multilingual thinking, at least to the extent of not automatically and routinely eliminating considerations from any of these perspectives. The problem at the same time is to avoid becoming a conceptual Tower of Babel. Such a multiaxial approach inevitably includes discrepant meanings for identical language. For example, from the perspective of biological interventions, "environmental manipulation" includes psychotherapy. When the focus is on psychological interventions, however, psychotherapy and environmental manipulation are conceived of as two distinctly different processes.

A more common result of this conceptual-linguistic versatility is the tendency to obscure essential similarities and areas of overlap. What happens is that different words and phrases that mean the same actually sound quite different because of their derivation from different schools of thought. In 1946 this was highlighted vividly by Witmer's *Psychiatric Interviews with Children* in which 10 child guidance cases are reported by nine psychotherapists representing different schools of psychotherapy. Witmer noted that the differences between the allegedly discrepant theoretical frames of reference faded out in actual clinical practice. Observing that the several therapists responded sensitively to the child's needs, Witmer asserted that certain principles basic to all child psychotherapy overshadowed the influence of the therapist's theoretical inclination.

Interrelationship of Behavioral and Psychodynamic Therapies

Perhaps we are currently observing a comparable phenomenon as it develops. During the 1960s there was a resurgence of interest in behavioral techniques, accompanied by an emphasis on the differences between behavioral and psychodynamic approaches. Eysenck (1960) stressed that treatment strategies that employ behavior explicitly should be distinguished from psychotherapy that employs psychological methods. A comparable segregationist attitude was as evident on the psychodynamic side where similar efforts to demarcate boundaries permeated the literature and educational programs. There was active depreciation of treatments that focused on symptoms; it was asserted, inaccurately as it happened but nevertheless dogmatically, that this could lead only to symptom substitution. Often enough there was a valid basis to this segregation, but too little attention was paid to the presence of psychological influences in even the most mechanistic behavioral techniques. The inevitable presence of behavioral influences in the "purest" psychological therapies was similarly ignored.

The exaggerated emphasis on this segregation has led to a tendency to neglect noteworthy integrationist efforts. Mowrer (1950) and Dollard and Miller (1950) endeavored to examine psychodynamic therapy from the perspective of learning-behavioral theory and were able to document cross-fertilization. More recently, there have been discussions of behavioral therapy with children from a psychodynamic perspective (e.g., Kessler, 1966; Blom, 1972). Feather (quoted by Aronson, 1972) suggested that some of the effectiveness of systematic desensitization in behavior therapy may be a consequence of enhancing the patient's discrimination between fantasy and reality. Contrariwise, the effectiveness of interpretation in psychoanalysis and related therapies may in part be derived from its desensitizing effect. There have been additional efforts (not focused on work with children) to synthesize these apparently conflicting perspectives, and to do this without minimizing, demeaning, or sacrificing the essential richness of the contribution of each point of view. Some of these have been made by Alexander (1963), Marks and Gelder (1966), Brady (1968), Sloane (1969), Lazarus (1969), Marmor (1971), and Feather and Rhoads (1972). In fact Marks (1971) has noted that even the term "behavior therapy," which seems so amenable to description and classification when compared to many of the other psychotherapies, has lost much of its meaning. Today it denotes a number of different techniques, many of which Marks asserts have little in common with one another beyond "common lip-service to debatable, theoretical antecedents." In his view, there are more differences than similarities between desensitization, aversion, operant conditioning, modeling, covert sensitization, feedback control, and negative practice. Further, he observes that flooding or implosion is considered to be a behavior therapy although it was originally conceived by Stampfl in psychodynamic terms; on the other hand, paradoxical intention, an allied technique, is thought of as a form of existential psychotherapy.

Probably the most vivid examples of integration of psychodynamic and behavioral approaches, even though they are not always explicitly seen as such, are to be found in the milieu therapy of child psychiatric residential and day treatment facilities. Noshpitz (1971) noted what he referred to as a "ping-pong effect" in residential treatment. Behavioral change is initiated in the residential setting while its repercussions are explored concurrently in individual psychotherapeutic sessions so that the action in one arena and the information stemming from it augment and illuminate what transpires in the other arena. A case reported by McDermott, Fraiberg, and Harrison (1968) vividly illustrates that what occurs in a residential milieu can enhance the understanding of the individual psychotherapist, and that what transpires in the individual psychotherapeutic sessions can contribute to the formulation of behavioral management techniques for the milieu. Blom (1972) noted that change is "capable of being accomplished both from the inside out and the outside in."

Some years ago the distinguished behavioral therapist Richard B. Stuart presented videotapes of his clinical work to the predominantly psychodynamically oriented child psychiatry staff of the University of Michigan's Children's Psychiatric Hospital. What ensued illustrated the rich potential of these interrelationships as well as their complexity. Although two apparently opposing views of the same therapeutic endeavor will be described below, it cannot be emphasized too much that the intent is not to underscore the correctness of one point of view by using the other as a straw man. The purpose is to illustrate that both perspectives can convey the impression of simultaneous validity and mutual incompatibility.

My recollection of that presentation was that Dr. Stuart began with charts quantifying the use of reinforcers and the appearance of specific undesirable behaviors, both of which rapidly decreased. The audience was much impressed with the correlation between the intervention and the behavioral results until we viewed the tapes.

The background of the videotapes was that Dr. Stuart had become acquainted with the family through the juvenile court, where several of the children had recent involvement because of minor delinquencies. All the manifest difficulties reportedly started shortly after the death of their father. He had been the nurturant, child-rearing, homemaking parent, whereas the mother was the breadwinner. His death had been sudden, occurring while several of the children were at home and the mother at work. After his death, all the children experienced varying degrees of difficulty in school and in the community. These problems overwhelmed the mother, whose only successful means of dealing with her children was to have a male neighbor paddle them. Such physical measures had not been used while the father was alive.

The taped therapeutic sessions were conducted in the family's home. The first sessions began chaotically with what sounded like several of the children's radios tuned loudly to different stations. Although the noise made it difficult to conceive of verbal communication, four-letter words were readily heard as shouting and interrupting prevailed. Meanwhile, the mother sat quietly, appearing apathetic, disheveled, and overwhelmed.

Making himself heard above the din, Dr. Stuart asked the youngsters to turn off their radios, after which he asserted that he would be working with the family on a regular basis to help them overcome their difficulties. As he realized that his assistance might be required in the interim between the scheduled meetings, he gave the mother and the children telephone numbers where he could be reached 24 hours a day. He then tried to determine their concept of their difficulties; the children described this as insufficient money, or items that money could buy. Although finances were not a substantial problem, the therapist responded by using money as a reinforcer. The children were to be rewarded with coins for avoiding certain undesirable behaviors, such as interrupting, talking rudely and disrespectfully to one another, swearing, and forcing others to shout by playing the radio loudly. The rewards were accompanied by what appeared to be the therapist's approval and he encouraged them to engage in interactions which could resolve some of the issues that were keeping them apart.

The videotapes of subsequent sessions confirmed the dramatic change in the children that had been demonstrated in the charts. The most striking change perceived by the audience, however, and one which had not been charted, was in the mother. She was now responsive to her children; she appeared alert and well groomed; and it was evident that she focused a great deal of attention on Dr. Stuart. He agreed that the change in the mother was striking, and he attributed it to two factors: the mother learned (or relearned) some assertive strategies of child-rearing, and the diminution of the children's negative behaviors and the increase in their positive behaviors reduced the pressure under which the mother lived. These changes resulted from Stuart's (1976, personal communication) employment of the three sets of skills which he conceives as necessary to effect therapeutic change. First are service-delivery skills, which increase the client's readiness to accept constructive suggestions. The second consists of behavior-change skills designed to alter focal behavior. Third are maintenance skills, which differ from those techniques which are needed to change the focal behavior in the first place. Instead, they are specifically designed to help the client anticipate and learn to deal with potential threats to the newly acquired changes.

In the tape and vignettes described above, Dr. Stuart perceived the service-delivery skills as including structuring the treatment environment, establishing a trustful relationship with the mother and the children, etc. The behavior-change skills included shaping constructive social interaction during the sessions and contracting for the predictable exchange of privileges and responsibilities between sessions. He summarized his view of the therapy illustrated on the tape as "an effort to model these techniques for the mother who is expected later to assume them herself."

Without necessarily assuming that any of Stuart's observations or formulations were incorrect, the psychodynamically oriented clinicians in the audience perceived them from a markedly different perspective. It was noted that the striking changes in the mother were neither charted nor otherwise highlighted, nor were these substantial alterations a consequence of any focal technology for promoting behavioral changes since none was directed toward her. Consequently, it was questioned whether there might be a factor operating that might have preceded her reaction to the marked changes in her children's behavior. For example, to what extent could the changes in the mother be a response to the therapist's 24-hour availability and the sensitivity of his courtly and respectful demeanor toward her, even when she appeared apathetic? We reasoned that the children's negative behavior may well have been an effort to evoke a response from this seemingly indifferent, uncaring mother, who had initially sat impassive and apathetic while the children bombarded her with epithets. It was recalled that earlier, when the mother had first tried to cope with the children, she had enlisted the aid of an outside man. Could it be that the mother's newfound responsiveness was secondary to the therapist's forceful participation with the family? More than that, when the mother responded to the therapist, had this diminished the children's need for outlandish behavior? The audience was impressed also with Dr. Stuart's sensitive handling of interactions within the family; he had worked in the manner of a highly skilled family therapist. Thus, this psychodynamically oriented audience perceived the behavioral reinforcement that had been so rigorously quantified and precisely charted as a relatively minor therapeutic intervention. In response, it was pointed out that a psychiatric resident, who presumably possessed service-delivery skills but lacked a mastery of focal technology designed to promote behavioral change, had previously attempted treatment without success. Nonetheless, these questions persisted.

Evolving Identity of Family Therapy

It is unwise to render historical judgments about developments that are still in process. Despite this, it seems safe to say that over the course of its brief two decades of productive activity, significant aspects of family therapy have become increasingly segregationist. It has been striving for a special identity, one that is not just another modality that a clinician can add to his roster of therapeutic options. Thus, there have been declarations that family therapy is a unique perspective on the human condition, one that is not conceptually interchangeable with other therapies. The argument goes further, casting away the medical model, disease concepts of emotional disturbance, and the individualistic and intrapsychic emphases in psychodynamic psychiatry. One may well question whether the maintenance of these increasingly impenetrable boundaries reflects insufficient distinction between the *study* of family processes and their *treatment*. It is easy to envision that the investigation of families would be enhanced by segregation of research in a manner analogous to a university's departmental structure, lending rigor and systematization to the area of study. On the other hand, therapy and the people seeking help are different from departments; they are generally enriched by integration.

The segregationist trend seems to be gaining momentum. One of its unfortunate by-products is that some child-oriented clinicians are apparently getting discouraged and are not benefiting from the fruitfulness of the family therapy field. At the same time there are encouraging indications. Integration of the systems-oriented transactional model with the developmental and psychodynamic models (e.g., Kramer, 1968) is expanding. McDermott and Char (1974) point out that systems theory, on the one hand, suggests that the sum of the parts does not explain the whole; but the converse is also true: knowledge of the whole family system does not necessarily entail understanding its parts, particularly the parts that are developing most rapidly. McDermott and Char recall that child psychiatry has struggled long and hard to establish that treating children's difficulties often requires more than counseling and treating parents. Malone (1974) discusses the advantages of flexibly combining therapeutic work with individuals, family subsystems, and total families. He asserts that the "central concept involved is the inseparability of internal and external." This strikes a chord reminiscent of Blom's (1972) observation about the interrelatability and interdependence of the behavioral and psychodynamic perspectives.

Pharmacotherapy and Psychotherapy

The issue of combining treatments that affect different aspects of the same difficulty in the same person is illustrated most vividly by the relationships between the psychotherapies and the pharmacotherapies. Over the past two decades, the proponents of each have been characterized by considerable competitiveness that has escalated into a mutually antagonistic exclusiveness. From a rational standpoint, it is self-evident that prescribing medication should not preclude attention to intrapsychic and interpersonal factors, nor should the use of psychotherapy necessarily preclude using medication or environmental intervention. Nevertheless, the proponents of each treatment modality have tended to view those of the other with suspicion and indignation, each group behaving as if the other did not exist while ritualistically giving lip service to one another. The choice of treatment method has stemmed more from the clinician's education, orientation, skills, preferences, etc. than from clinical indications and demonstrated effectiveness.

As increasing numbers of physicians have been exposed to the theory and practice of both psychotherapy and pharmacotherapy, the competition between the two has been diminishing and they are more and more being judiciously employed together. Nevertheless, a scholarly GAP report (1975) devoted to the paradoxes, problems, and progress in the interrelationships between pharmacotherapy and psychotherapy notes that such physicians remain unable to translate psychological conflict into cellular malfunction, or biochemical dysfunction into behavioral difficulties. As a result the physicians often behave like "split-brain preparations," comfortable only with one frame of reference at a time and experiencing difficulty with the simultaneous use of both frames of reference. There is a lack of coherent integrating theory, or even of interrelating hypotheses, to combine what is known psychodynamically with what is known psychopharmacologically. Mandell (1976) has labeled the need to forget psychodynamics selectively while prescribing psychotropic medication the "peek-a-boo" use of drugs. One hopes that this will diminish as a consequence of a number of promising contributions. An example is Gittelman-Klein and Klein's (1973) study of imipramine's effect on youngsters who refused to go to school. From this they derived the concept that tricyclics reduce primary separation anxiety without affecting anticipatory anxiety.

Universal Concepts

Certain concepts are basic to almost every therapeutic transaction. This phenomenon makes it possible for truly different treatment modalities to be related. Although operant reinforcement is, for example, part of behavioral-learning theory, it is hard to conceive of any therapeutic transaction to which this concept would not be applicable. Similarly, such psychoanalytic and/or psychodynamic concepts as transference and countertransference merit serious consideration in exclusively pharmacologic or behavioral therapeutic interactions. Indeed, it is likely that the operant reinforcement employed by the clinician and the manner in which he or she deals with the patient's transference reactions are significant, if not central, in shaping the nature of every therapy.

SELECTING THE APPROPRIATE TREATMENT

A 1973 GAP report devoted to child psychiatric treatment planning outlined five cases of school refusal (pp. 604-606). In each instance, diagnostic assessment led to a rational selection of five different therapeutic methods, each designed to change a different aspect of the child's existence. Their prime targets for change were either intrapsychic modification, alteration of intrafamilial functioning, alteration of peer-group interaction, modification of the child's school or community adjustment, or temporary removal of the child to a different environment.

To underscore the value of selective therapeutic differentiation based on diagnostic considerations, additional syndromes and clinical examples will be cited in the following sections.

Hyperactivity

Currently, perhaps the most prominent clinical symptom in children for which there is no standard unitary therapeutic approach is hyperactivity. The hyperactivity might represent a means for expressing or discharging anxiety resulting from an unconscious intrapsychic conflict over aggression. In such an instance, the treatment of choice at child psychiatry's current level of knowledge would be antianxiety medication to suppress the symptom and/or interpretive psychotherapy to resolve the child's conflicts. On the other hand, if the hyperactivity is a consequence of minimal brain dysfunction, the clinician will endeavor to provide externally the controls that the youngster lacks internally. To do so may require a combination of stimulant medication and regulation of the child's life via supportive-suppressive measures (such as helping the child learn to isolate himself from distressing stimuli).

These different therapeutic approaches to a hyperactive youngster are not truly interchangeable. When the hyperactivity stems from underlying anxiety, regulating the child's life may indeed diminish the symptom, but the symptom relief is likely to be accomplished at the cost of inducing passivity as a means of handling the unconscious aggression. In other words, the inappropriate treatment might seem to be effective because it induces a new and unnecessary handicap that proves to be less troublesome to parents and teachers. When the hyperactivity is a consequence of organicity and the child is offered psychotherapeutic interpretations regarding underlying conflicts, these interpretations tend to be stimulating and may well cause the child to become excited and more hyperactive. In fact, this may be accentuated by the accuracy of the interpretations because it is not the underlying psychological conflicts that are primarily pathogenic so much as the deficiency in internal controls.

The foregoing therapeutic approaches to hyperactivity focus exclusively on the individual child. Despite the fact that the treatment may be both appropriate and effective, it may serve to perpetuate the hyperactivity! This occurs when a family's stability and well-being have come to depend on the hyperactive child's behaving disruptively (irrespective of the etiology of the hyperactivity). For instance, some parents never go out because they allegedly need to be with their children constantly in order to control difficulties created by the hyperactive child. This may, in fact, be a way to avoid confronting painful marital difficulties. By tying themselves to their children, the parents are protected from being alone, and they can maintain their marital alliance by perceiving the hyperactive child as a common "enemy" about whom they invariably agree. Siblings, too, can maintain their own sense of self-esteem by assigning the cause of all arguments and fights to the obviously difficult hyperactive youngster. Such scapegoating may be identified by the clinical observation that one or both parents become depressed when treatment helps the youngster improve his behavior. Another hint comes when the clinician tries to focus on the parents' attitudes toward anger and finds that his efforts are invariably sidetracked by the parents' soliciting counseling for complicated child-management problems. A diagnostic family session may reveal siblings referring to the hyperactive youngster as "hyper-dummy" or similar appellations that seem to be accepted casually by the entire family. In such situations a family-therapeutic approach would be indicated either as the sole treatment or in conjunction with one or several of the aforementioned modalities.

It should be emphasized that this discussion is not a comprehensive statement regarding the possible causes and treatment for hyperkinesis in children. Such an account would require review of the possible influences of allergies, intolerance of food additives, carbohydrate imbalance, insecticides, lead poisoning, fluorescent lighting, etc. The intent is rather to illustrate the general point about the selection of treatment methods.

Learning Disorders

Another common clinical problem is that of the child suffering from learning impairment. In planning intervention for such cases, it is important to determine whether the academic difficulties are caused by developmental arrest, undefended regression, or psychological inhibitions. The treatment of choice for the child with developmental arrest is remedial education. But, for children whose therapeutic need is the reversal of regression or the exposure of intrapsychic conflicts to consciousness, such an approach may prove to be utterly futile. This type of therapeutic misapplication tends to occur as a consequence of failure to penetrate beyond the phenomenologic level in assessment. It can prove harmful as well as merely futile. The youngster with reading retardation secondary to underlying emotional factors who does not respond to tutoring is likely to take this failure as further evidence of his stupidity and hopelessness. Thus, regardless of how enthusiastically it is pursued, if the therapeutic effort neglects the underlying cause, it may well reinforce the symptom. In addition, albeit unwittingly, such efforts may repeat a significant trauma. For example:

> In his three years of schooling, eight-year-old John was unable even to begin to learn the alphabet. Intensive tutoring had been ineffective, and subsequent psychotherapy revealed that the tutoring had in fact increased his resistance to learning. During the course of psychotherapy, it emerged that John's sister, three years his senior, used to play school with him. This game had started when she was five and he was two. She played the role of teacher, and John and some dolls were the pupils. His inability to learn the alphabet in this game prompted his five-year-old teacher to be threatening and punitive. Harshly, she warned John repeatedly that he would never be permitted to attend school unless he learned. This frightening game and the warnings persisted until John entered school. Reconstruction in psychotherapy showed that John was sure he would dread and hate school. Unconsciously, he was determined not to learn, so that he would be denied entry into school. Only after uncovering and working through these experiences and their associated ideas, feelings, and attitudes was he able to dismiss them as inappropriate to his actual school situation and for the first time to benefit from tutoring. Until that point, he had unconsciously viewed tutoring as a punishment that reinforced his determination not to learn from it (Harrison, 1975).

DIFFERENT METHODS AT VARIOUS PHASES OF TREATMENT

Therapeutic intervention requires a capacity for effective problem-solving in complex situations. The problem is usually multidimensional, of mixed etiology, with the idiosyncratic features of the individual and/or family always present. As a bio-psycho-social synthesis, a person suffering disturbance in one aspect of the integrated human system often experiences it as being reflected in other parts of the system. Thus, the system manifesting the most disturbance is not necessarily the one in which the basic problem resides. Similarly, the fact that a therapy directed to a particular system is effective does not necessarily constitute evidence that the primary difficulty is located there; e.g., for a given hyperactive youngster, the effectiveness of methylphenidate is not in itself proof of a chemical or organic etiology. Consequently, clinicians are inevitably faced with the interesting challenge of systemic interrelationships which demand multifaceted therapeutic modes. The following case illustrates the use of different therapeutic approaches at various phases of the clinical work with the same child and family.

Eight-year-old Carol was displaying unsatisfactory academic progress and a lack of peer relationships. Both her third-grade teacher and the school psychologist urged her divorced mother to seek psychiatric help for her. Carol's unhappiness was evident in her demeanor and verbalization, as well as in her tendency to hang around school long after dismissal, seeking out male teachers and the male janitor. Although her mother had not perceived the difficulties, she cooperated in a psychiatric evaluation. She accepted a recommendation for Carol to enter individual psychodynamically oriented exploratory psychotherapy. The goal was to facilitate working through unresolved feelings about the parental divorce. The mother simultaneously participated in a combination of parent counseling and therapy designed to help her shaky self-concept and inconsistent parenting.

The same therapist saw Carol twice a week and the mother weekly for more than a year; both mother and daughter made considerable progress. Mother had always allowed others to dominate her, but she now stood up for what she believed to be right. She was evidently a far more effective person, with an enhanced self-concept as a parent. With the notable exception of peer relationships which were limited to her siblings or very young neighbor children, Carol's accomplishments were evident in all other areas.

At this point the therapist elected to add focal family therapy to the therapeutic program. This added a third modality to the other two interrelated treatments. The rationale for this stemmed from the following: Carol's birth as the youngest and only female of four natural children had been eagerly awaited by her parents. Her mother recalled with considerable warmth the closeness that she shared with Carol as an infant; this was maintained until around age two when Carol's efforts toward autonomy assumed an oppositional negativistic flavor. This posed considerable difficulty for her parents, who proposed and implemented an unusual solution. They adopted a same-aged sister for Carol, ostensibly to provide her with companionship. The clinical work with the mother suggested that the parents' un-conscious motivation was to bludgeon Carol back into being an obedient little baby by providing her with a model of correct behavior. Thus, when Carol was two and a half, Charlene, who was also two and a half, joined the family. Apparently spurred by her own need to establish herself in the family in the face of insecure feelings about adoption, Charlene readily assumed the assigned role of the model child. Over the years she developed into the perfect daughter while Carol, by contrast, appeared stupid and remained immature and vulnerable.

The individual therapeutic work illuminated the strong mutual identification between mother and biological daughter. The mother's inadequate self-concept stemmed substantially from perceiving herself as having always been a disappointment to her own father. The successful working through in therapy of this oedipal disappointment enabled mother to change her attitudes toward her daughter. Simultaneously, in her own work with the therapist, Carol dealt with competitive feelings for her sister. The family interaction, however, continued to encourage Carol to be the inadequate little girl while Charlene kept the role of the capable model. In the face of these external familial factors, the therapist's efforts to resolve Carol's intrapsychic internalized self-concept proved insufficient. Carol continued to maintain this "little" attitude. Charlene persisted in her successfully competitive attitude toward Carol. For instance, on those occasions when Carol would venture to bring a friend home, Charlene would successfully take the friend away from Carol.

The focal family therapy served to identify those external pressures on Carol and endeavored to make them family-dystonic. To some extent this relieved Carol of the "identified-patient" scapegoat role by making her shortcomings a family problem as well as her own. Simultaneously, an effort was made to relieve Charlene's need to maintain a place in the family by being superior. During the family therapy it became evident that Charlene's security within the family was vulnerable, not only because of her adopted status, but also because of the extrusion of the divorced father, Charles, with whom Charlene shared other qualities besides the similarity in names.

CLINICIAN'S USE OF SELF

For the same clinician to treat Carol with individual exploratory psychotherapy, to undertake a combination of parent counseling and personal psychotherapy with her mother, and to engage the entire family in focal family therapy requires a degree of dexterity in the clinician's use of self that may not be within the capacity of all child psychiatrists. It is incumbent on clinicians to be cognizant of their capabilities and limitations in this regard. Despite all the advances in psychopharmacology and in therapeutic use of the behavioral, social, milieu, and other external agents and instruments, the clinician's personality remains a potent and important diagnostic and therapeutic instrument. Many psychiatric treatments are enhanced by a quality of spontaneity on the part of the therapist. Indeed, except in the biological and some of the behavioral therapies, the therapist has limited opportunity to calculate the dosage of each therapeutic intervention. In consequence, once they have assessed the situation and determined their approach, experienced therapists generally behave quite spontaneously. These quasi "spontaneous" therapeutic interventions are then subjected to post hoc scrutiny and critical review. Child psychiatric work, therefore, encompasses individualistic styles of practice that require the clinician to achieve a considerable degree of self-understanding, self-realization, and self-actualization. These capacities in turn encourage the refinement of his sensitivity, empathy, and intuition. Such traits are central to the participant-observer combination of evocative listening and intervention that characterizes almost all of the diagnostic assessments and so many of the therapeutic interventions of the mental health professional.

Child psychiatrists are well aware that the use of self calls for a change in the detached-approach model that characterizes most other types of medical practice. During their residency many have observed that accomplishing this change may require substantial alterations in their previously adequate coping styles. This is one area for which educational programs typically offer little help. In addition, different clinical approaches tend to require further differentiation in use of self.

Many psychodynamically oriented approaches postulate that the patient changes via cognitive-affective reexperiencing of the introjected past. This takes place in the course of a special kind of encounter with the therapist. To achieve this, the clinician is taught to keep personal reactions under control while observing his own internal processes. His goal is to discriminate between objective professional reactions, reactions stemming from his own past, and reactions stimulated by the patient. Meanwhile, the patient is encouraged to look at himself, to explore the past and to study its effect on the present. The result is a deep and powerful interaction that can approach aspects of the religious-magical contact between shaman and client. It places enormous demands on the therapist who in a sense experiences the patient through himself as though the therapist were a part of the other's phenomenology.

In contrast, by incorporating a more naturalistic and scientific mode, the biologic and behavioral therapies do not burden the therapist with the same requirements. Indeed, they encourage the clinician to distance himself from the patient in an effort to maximize objectivity. Prediction and control of the problem are emphasized at the expense of understanding the patient's subjective experience.

A systems orientation and the related social intervention modes such as family therapy postulate that change stems from the therapist's affiliation with the family (or other social system). He uses his relationship to alter individual roles in the dysfunctional transactional processes of the family and in its total structural organization. In contrast to the psychodynamic, biologic, and behavioral modes, the clinician is usually taught not to guard against spontaneous personal responses. It is assumed that those responses will be system-syntonic; even if they are not, they can serve as valuable exploratory probes. The therapist's spontaneity contributes to establishing an affiliation with the family and experiencing its pressures.

QUALITIES REQUIRED FOR THERAPEUTIC DIFFERENTIATION

It is inevitable that clinicians will be far more competent in some intervention modes than in others. With the passage of time, it becomes increasingly difficult for individual clinicians to be so versatile that they are knowledgeable and expert in all the available types of child psychiatric treatment. As it is no longer easy to be "Renaissance" therapists, it is incumbent on the practitioner to be alert to and avoid the temptation to limit therapeutic recommendations to those modalities with which he is most familiar. The child psychiatrist is a psychosocially oriented human biologist with a special skill in diagnostic assessment and multidimensional formulation of the problem. He has to be prepared to prescribe a wide range of therapeutic interventions in a knowledgeable and selective fashion.

The ability to consider the broad range of possible treatments and the readiness to do so are prerequisites for a comprehensive diagnostic assessment. These do not, however, have to be extended as far as the actual administration of the therapy. Indeed, in treating patients, it is often advantageous to tune out selectively those techniques judged to be inappropriate for the particular patient or family. Not only are many techniques contraindicated in a specific situation but endeavoring to keep the related ideas in mind would risk creating the aforementioned Tower of Babel. Therefore, the initial diagnostic assessment and the reassessments during the course of therapy require broad-gauged professional competence, but the actual administration of the treatment does not. Indeed, a limited focus may enhance the quality of the treatment.

It is evident that other professionals and/or paraprofessionals are becoming skilled in specific delimited therapies. This tends to threaten those child psychiatrists who only yesteryear were the most expert at everything and draped themselves in an aura of clinical omnipotence. It has required adaptation to accept the fact that nurses and child-care workers may be far more expert in life-space interviewing, and that a paraprofessional inner-city resident is more gifted at talking down the drug-overdosed, acutely psychotic adolescent. A variety of factors have enabled child psychiatrists to adjust to such situations, but would the same be true for such sophisticated and elitist techniques as psychoanalytic therapy?

Such demarcations of expertise are accepted comfortably by many child psychiatrists in other countries. Concern about it is primarily an American phenomenon, often accompanied by a tendency to think of psychiatry in other nations as inferior. There is evidence of a diminution of this superior attitude; this may be associated with modification of the previously overwhelming influence of the psycho-dynamic point of view.

Other medical specialists have also adapted to sharing health-care delivery with others who have greater expertise in well-defined areas. Consider the ophthalmologist vis à vis the optician and, increasingly, the optometrist. Another example is the orthopedist vis à vis the physical therapist and brace maker.

Yet, the ophthalmologist, orthopedist, and others have retained exclusive expertise in what tends to be universally perceived as the most significant aspect of the activity. In child psychiatry, however, diagnostic assessments, treatment planning, prescription, coordination, and reassessment have not always been considered the most esteemed aspects of the work.

Advocating that child psychiatrists should be familiar with the wide array of available treatment methods as a prerequisite for our seminal problem-solving responsibility should be carefully distinguished from being truly knowledgeable and expert in applying these methods. The intent is for the child psychiatrist to be a complete clinician. The general physician must be familiar with insulin for diabetic coma and craniotomy for intracranial pathology in order to deal with the comatose patient. This is true even though he is not personally capable of administering all these forms of treatment. Does this entail a potential for a little knowledge to be dangerous? Obviously, if clinicians believe they are expert in areas in which they possess only a degree of familiarity, this would be inconsistent with responsible professionalism. Becoming familiar with intervention modes about which they know little should enhance clinicians' capacity to assess with greater precision where their expertise begins and ends. This should help also to achieve greater freedom from rigid adherence to any preferred theoretical model of human development and deviance, and should allow the clinician to reach beyond the therapeutic interventions related to such a preferred framework. In the absence of such autonomy, the child psychiatrist risks confining himself to a limited therapeutic range which deals with only one aspect of the psychobiosocial system.

None of the emphasis here on a multidimensional pluralistic integration is intended to deny that there are clinical situations in which a unitary approach is best. Thus, a careful clinical assessment may suggest that for a given case an exclusive, rigidly adhered to therapeutic strategy is indicated for a particular youngster and/or family. Here, however, the intention is to assert that by and large children do not get better because child psychiatrists display an unvarying devotion to a particular technique with all patients, a devotion to which the various mental health fields seem to be exquisitely vulnerable. This is especially true when interest is building up around an exciting new therapeutic strategy. Some clinicians react to new developments by shutting their eyes to the new approaches and clinging tenaciously to what they have always done. Other clinicians may be readily persuaded to join the enthusiastic proponents of the new method who write and speak to the point of overzealousness about the merits of exclusive use of a particular treatment. That seems to have been the case with psychoanalysis in the 1940s and 1950s, whereas in the 1960s and 1970s similar claims are made for behavior therapy and family therapy.

Child psychiatry has much to learn about prescribing treatment. The goal is specificity and therapeutic differentiation, and the method by which to achieve these is based on meticulous diagnostic assessment. There is so much more to be learned about when nonspecific factors help; when the therapist's interest or charisma is all that is required; and when it is essential for children to have the benefit of specific psychological, behavioral, physiologic and/or environmental interventions. Perhaps the most important need is to learn when, in fact, nothing additional is needed to enhance the child's developmental potential. This knowledge can be accumulated only by methodologically sound, rigorously executed investigations that will document publicly the value of differentiated application of specific therapeutic interventions.

REFERENCES

ACKERMAN, N. W. 1958. *The Psychodynamics of Family Life.* New York: Basic Books.
ADAMS, P. L. 1974. *A Primer of Child Psychotherapy.* Boston: Little, Brown.
ALEXANDER, F. 1963. The dynamics of therapy in the light of learning theory. *Am. J. Psychiatry,* 120:440-448.

ARONSON, G. 1972. Learning theory and psychoanalytic theory. *J. Am. Psychoanal. Assoc.*, 20:622-637.

BETTELHEIM, B., and SYLVESTER, E. 1948. A therapeutic milieu. *Am. J. Orthopsychiatry*, 18:191-206.

BETTELHEIM, B., and SYLVESTER, E. 1949. Milieu therapy—indications and illustrations. *Psychoanal. Rev.*, 36:54-67.

BLOM, G. E. 1972. A psychoanalytic viewpoint of behavior modification in clinical and educational settings. *J. Am. Acad. Child Psychiatry*, 11:675-693.

BRADLEY, C. 1937. The behavior of children receiving benzedrine. *Am. J. Psychiatry*, 94:577-585.

BRADY, J. P. 1968. Psychotherapy by a combined behavioral and dynamic approach. *Compr. Psychiatry*, 9:536-543.

COHEN, R. L., RAFFERTY, F. T., ADAMS, P. L., MALONE, C. A., MARINE, E., BEACH, W. B., BERLIN, I. N., SONIS, M., and SONIS, A. C. 1975. Child psychiatric programs and the community mental health movement: A progress report. *J. Am. Acad. Child Psychiatry*, 14:1-113.

DOLLARD, J., and MILLER, N. 1950. *Personality and Psychotherapy*. New York: McGraw-Hill.

EYSENCK, H. J. 1960. *Behavior Therapy and the Neuroses: Readings and Modern Methods of Treatment Derived from Learning Theory*. Elmsford, N.Y.: Pergamon Press.

FEATHER, B. W., and RHOADS, J. M. 1972. Psychodynamic behavior therapy. *Arch. Gen. Psychiatry*, 26:496-511.

FERENCZI, S. 1913. A little chanticleer. In *Contributions of Psychoanalysis*. New York: Robert Brunner, 1950.

FRANK, J. 1961. *Persuasion and Healing*. Baltimore: Johns Hopkins University Press.

FREUD, S. 1909. Analysis of a phobia in a five-year-old boy. In *Standard Edition of the Complete Psychological Works of Sigmund Freud*, 1955, vol. 10, pp. 1-49. London: Hogarth Press.

GITTELMAN-KLEIN, R., and KLEIN, D. F. 1973. School phobia: Diagnostic considerations in the light of imipramine effects. *J. Nerv. Ment. Dis.*, 156:199-215.

GROUP FOR THE ADVANCEMENT OF PSYCHIATRY. 1962. *The Preclinical Teaching of Psychiatry*. Report No. 54. New York: Group for the Advancement of Psychiatry.

GROUP FOR THE ADVANCEMENT OF PSYCHIATRY. 1966. *Psychopathological Disorders in Childhood: Theoretical Considerations and a Proposed Classification*, vol. 6, Report No. 6, pp. 173-343. New York: Group for the Advancement of Psychiatry.

GROUP FOR THE ADVANCEMENT OF PSYCHIATRY. 1973. *From Diagnosis to Treatment: An Approach to Treatment Planning for the Emotionally Disturbed Child*, vol. 8, Report No. 87, pp. 520-661. New York: Group for the Advancement of Psychiatry.

GROUP FOR THE ADVANCEMENT OF PSYCHIATRY. 1975. *Pharmacotherapy and Psychotherapy: Paradoxes, Problems and Progress*, vol. 9, Report No. 93, pp. 261-431. New York: Group for the Advancement of Psychiatry.

HALLECK, S., and WOODS, S. 1962. Emotional problems of psychiatric residents. *Psychiatry*, 25:339-346.

HARRISON, S. I. 1975. Individual psychotherapy. In A. M. Freedman, H. I. Kaplan, and B. J. Sadock (eds.), *Comprehensive Textbook of Psychiatry*—II, chapter 40.1, pp. 2214-2228. Baltimore: Williams & Wilkins.

HARRISON, S. I., and CAREK, D. J. 1966. *A Guide to Psychotherapy*. Boston: Little, Brown.

HUG-HELLMUTH, H. V. 1921. On the technique of child analysis. *Int. J. Psychoanal.*, 2:287-305.

JONES, M. 1953. *The Therapeutic Community*. New York: Basic Books.
JONES, M. C. 1924. The elimination of children's fears. *J. Exp. Psychol.*, 7:382-390.
KESSLER, J. W. 1966. *Psychopathology of Childhood*. Englewood Cliffs, N.J.: Prentice-Hall.
KETY, S. S. 1960. The true nature of a book: An allegory. *NIH Record*, June 7, 1960.
KLAGSBRUN, S. 1967. In search of an identity. *Arch. Gen. Psychiatry*, 16:286-289.
KRAMER, C. H. 1968. *Psychoanalytically Oriented Family Therapy: Ten Year Evolution in a Private Child Psychiatry Practice*. Monograph. Family Institute of Chicago.
LAZARUS, A. A. 1969. Behavior therapy in graded structure. *International Psychiatric Clinics*, 6:134-143.
LUBORSKY, L., SINGER, E., and LUBORSKY, L. 1975. Comparative studies of psychotherapies. *Arch. Gen. Psychiatry*, 32:995-1008.
MALONE, C. A. 1974. Observations on the role of family therapy in child psychiatry training. *J. Am. Acad. Child Psychiatry*, 13:437-458.
MANDELL, A. J. 1976. Dr. Hunter S. Thompson and a new psychiatry. *Psychiatry Digest*, 37 (3):12-17.
MARKS, I. 1971. The future of the psychotherapies. *Br. J. Psychiatry*, 118:69-72.
MARKS, I. M., and GELDER, M. G. 1966. Common ground between behavior therapy and psychodynamic methods. *Br. J. Med. Psychol.*, 39:11-23.
MARMOR, J. 1971. Dynamic psychotherapy and behavior therapy. *Arch. Gen. Psychiatry*, 24:22-28.
McDERMOTT, J. F., and CHAR, W. F. 1974. The undeclared war between child and family therapy. *J. Am. Acad. Child Psychiatry*, 13:422-436.
McDERMOTT, J. F., FRAIBERG, S., and HARRISON, S. I. 1968. Residential treatment of children: The utilization of transference behavior. *J. Am. Acad. Child Psychiatry*, 7:169-192.
MOWRER, O. H. 1950. *Learning Theory in Personality Dynamics*. New York: Ronald Press.
MOWRER, O. H., and MOWRER, W. 1938. Enuresis: A method for its study and treatment. *Am. J. Orthopsychiatry*, 8:436-459.
NOSHPITZ, J. D. 1971. The psychotherapist in residential treatment. In M. F. Mayer and A. Blum (eds.), *Healing Through Living: Symposium on Residential Care*. Springfield, Ill.: Thomas.
PIAGET, J. 1932. *The Moral Judgment of the Child*. London: Rutledge and Kegan Paul.
RESEARCH TASK FORCE OF THE NATIONAL INSTITUTE OF MENTAL HEALTH. 1975. *Research in the Service of Mental Health*. Rockville, Maryland: National Institute of Mental Health.
RUTTER, M., LEBOVICI, S., EISENBERG, L., SNEZREVSKIJ, A. V., SADOUN, R., BROOKE, E., and LIN, T. Y. 1969. A tri-axial classification of mental disorders in childhood: An international study. *J. Child Psychol. Psychiatry*, 10:41-61.
SLOANE, R. B. 1969. The converging paths of behavior therapy and psychotherapy. *Int. J. Psychiatry*, 7:493-503.
WATSON, J. B., and RAYNOR, R. 1920. Conditional emotional reactions. *J. Exp. Psychol.*, 3:1-14.
WITMER, H. L. 1946. *Psychiatric Interviews with Children*. New York: Commonwealth Fund.

7

What Adolescent Delinquents Taught Me About Psychotherapy Research

MILTON F. SHORE, Ph.D.

There are three ways to approach therapeutic intervention research with children and youth. One is to try to bring a new perspective to the vast literature on research on psychotherapy in general, and discuss how it might relate to the investigation of psychotherapeutic work with children. However, thorough analyses of psychotherapy research have been done recently, for instance in the large volume by Bergin and Garfield (1971), and the books by Meltzoff and Kornreich (1970), and Bergin and Strupp (1972). Therefore, it would be presumptuous to try to undertake such a task in a short article, if indeed it could be done at all.

A second approach is to bewail the amount or quality of research on child psychotherapy and to focus on the unique problems conceptually, methodologically, and in such areas as measurement from which one could derive some criteria for undertaking research in the child therapy area. But Heinicke and Strassmann (1975) have recently done a thorough and comprehensive review of child therapy research, and they have listed those criteria that should be met if one is to do good research on the effects of psychotherapy on children and youth.

The opinions expressed are those of the author and do not necessarily reflect the opinions or official position of the National Institute of Mental Health or the Department of Health, Education, and Welfare. Since the author is a government employee, this chapter is not covered by copyright.

A third approach, the one which I shall take, is to describe my own research with adolescent delinquents, the challenge and opportunities it offered, what it taught me about psychotherapy research, and how some of the problems that arise in the evaluation of the effectiveness of a new psychotherapeutic program were dealt with.

In order to highlight certain issues, I have divided this paper into five parts:

    I. Beyond Eysenck.
   II. The fruitless search for the familiar and simple independent variable.
  III. The wish for easy ways to measure complex change.
  IV. Does change wash out over time?
   V. So what does this tell us about people?

I. BEYOND EYSENCK

Eysenck's provocative article (1952) continues to be used by many critics of psychotherapy, particularly the advocates of behavior therapy, as evidence that psychotherapy has no effect. But, as might be expected, the field has developed rapidly over 25 years. No longer do we ask the broad and vague question, "Is psychotherapy effective?" We now more appropriately inquire: Psychotherapy for whom? What kind of psychotherapy? What is meant by "effective?"

Our program for adolescent delinquents began from a particular need. Although child psychiatry had many historical roots in treatment for delinquent youth, with outstanding figures such as Healy and Aichorn contributing to our understanding of antisocial behavior, child psychiatrists over the years have tended to become less involved with young people who have severe, long-standing antisocial behavioral problems. Meanwhile, a group of adolescent delinquents has developed that are more and more often being labeled "unreachable" or "untreatable" because they have not been helped by the standard methods of service delivery. These youngsters show early severe problems with school and legal authorities. By the time they reach 16 years of age, the legal age for leaving school, they have either been suspended or expelled, or have chosen to drop out on their

birthday (in reality the school has subtly encouraged them to leave).
Unlike the neurotic delinquent, they are viewed as having minimal
anxiety and long-standing characterological problems. When efforts
have been made to reach these youngsters, they have often appeared
for one or two interviews and left, never to return for help.

The aim of the work I shall describe was to develop a new way
of working with these so-called "unreachable" young people and to
determine whether our technique was effective (Massimo and Shore,
1963). To make certain we had a homogeneous group, we developed precise criteria for selection, purposely eliminating adolescents
who were neurotic, psychotic, brain-damaged, or mentally defective.
Programs for these groups would require different techniques from
those we planned. In other words, we developed a technique designed
to help a specific group in a specific way based on our understanding
of the nature of the difficulty, an understanding derived from psychoanalytic theory and from crisis theory, as well as from our unsuccessful efforts to help this group over many years.

Our selection criteria were specific: Age 15 to 17; IQ above 85
on a standard intelligence scale; a long history of antisocial behavior
with repeated truancy; long-standing problems in school adjustment
and performance; overt aggression toward peers and authority; a
reputation known to school attendance officers, courts, and the police;
suspension or expulsion from school or voluntary dropping out because of poor school performance and antisocial behavior; no grossly
observable psychotic behavior, and no previous psychotherapy for
the boy or members of his family that lasted for more than one
month.

The program that evolved, based on our clinical knowledge and
experience, had 10 elements. In an effort to give it a name, we called
it "comprehensive vocationally oriented psychotherapy" (Massimo
and Shore, 1967). The elements were:

1. Contact with the youth was initiated at a crisis point—when the
boy was expelled or suspended, or had dropped out of school. It was
believed that leaving school was a crisis and, therefore, according to

crisis theory, made the youth more amenable to help. Each boy was contacted within 24 hours after leaving school.

2. The initial approach to the boy was in terms of help in getting a job. Other possibilities like assistance with personal problems or getting a driver's license were merely mentioned as available if desired. This was based on our experience that these antisocial young people reject any program labeled as psychotherapy or academic help, but are often motivated to some degree to find a job. Our experience had also indicated that unless there was a meaningful, concrete goal in the first interview, these youths were not likely to appear for more than one session. Finding a job, therefore, was a precise and, to some degree, meaningful task to them.

3. Preemployment counseling focused on job readiness. To assist the antisocial youth in getting and keeping a job, his expectations and attitudes with regard to work were explored. Jobs were not preselected, but found in response to identified needs of the individual youth.

4. Following the outreach part of the program when initial contact was made, the self-initiating individualized aspects of the program were stressed. No part was rigidly defined. Focus was on the youth's responsibility for making decisions. In this way, the dependency, which we believed these antisocial youths characteristically fear and which sometimes is encouraged in many psychotherapeutic situations, was not fostered.

5. Flexibility of technique was maintained. There were minimal time restrictions and few limits on the contacts or activities of the therapist. Rigidity was avoided. Techniques varied with the demands of the immediate situation. The therapist spoke with or saw the youth any time of day or night and as often as 8 or 10 times a week, sometimes for many hours.

6. Motility and action were emphasized. The therapist had no central office. Field trips were taken frequently. In essence, the therapist played many roles and entered all areas of the youth's life—job-

finding, court appearances, pleasure trips, driving lessons when needed, locating or obtaining a car, arranging dentist appointments, going for glasses, shopping for clothes with first paycheck, opening a bank account, and other activities. These activities were done with the youth in such a way as to encourage mastery, not foster dependency.

7. The independence of the service from school, hospital, courts, or other social or authoritarian agencies was emphasized. The therapist was in no way involved in influencing the court's decisions on these boys or the decision of an employer to keep or fire a boy. Instead, all these events became part of the therapeutic intervention. Return-to-school overtures were not made. It was discovered that there were many alternatives to the public school program such as on-the-job training, night courses, or correspondence courses that these young people found useful in their work.

8. Treatment focused on individual responsibility, not group activity or participation. Support was constantly available, always on a one-to-one basis.

9. The remedial education program was tailored to individual needs and initially was closely related to work performance. It was initiated when the youth was ready to seek such assistance to improve his skills on the job.

10. After placement on a job, focus in psychotherapy shifted from job readiness to the problems encountered at work and in the community. Reality situations were used as modes for communicating psychotherapeutic insights.

The program lasted 10 months. Each youth was aware of the fact that this program would end after the 10 months.

II. THE FRUITLESS SEARCH FOR THE FAMILIAR AND SIMPLE INDEPENDENT VARIABLE

As can be seen from the description, the program for these antisocial youths differed from classical psychotherapy. This has resulted in some criticism. A well-known proponent of behavior modification rejected the intervention as psychotherapy because it dealt with a general social problem, rather than a personal neurotic disturbance. Researchers have asked, "What brought about change—Was it the job placement? The academic tutoring? The interpretations of pathological behavior?" A psychoanalyst in London attacked it as "just a Big Brother approach," although unfortunately, few Big Brothers are able to intervene appropriately and successfully with such an extremely disturbed group of youths without special training in psychotherapy like that received by the therapist in this program. Some psychoanalysts have felt uncomfortable because there was little personal history on these youths, although many of us would question the validity of any information given by this particular group of young people, as well as the general relevance of much of the historical material obtained in psychotherapeutic intervention with adolescents.

All these critics seemed to be searching for something that would easily fit into their characteristic way of working. Many were also searching for a simple, clear-cut intervention technique, a simple independent variable like those found in the scientific laboratory. Such a search, however, is fruitless and unnecessarily limiting when one deals with the pervasive problems and needs that groups like our chronic antisocial adolescents had.

Psychotherapy with children and youths challenges our conceptual ingenuity because it requires a broader view of the dimensions and techniques of intervention and of the elements that go into producing behavioral change. The inclusion of parents in treatment, the role of education, the role of maturation, the effects of all institutions on a child's life, the therapist's involvement as a real person in real-life situations, all pose major problems for how one defines the agent of change. It becomes clear, however, that what we need is a broader, rather than narrower, conceptual framework when we study intervention with children and youths. Such a larger view does not reduce the validity of the intervention. The validity and appropriateness of intervention come not from trying to define discrete and often mechanistic elements, as some might lead us to believe, but from being able to describe (even in general terms) what is being done, to train others to do it, and then to determine clearly if what was expected was indeed accomplished. It is my belief that the search for the elusive and unattainable simple variable of intervention has been one cause of the ever-widening gap between researcher and therapist and has led to a general avoidance and distrust of research on psychotherapeutic intervention with children.

III. THE WISH FOR EASY WAYS TO MEASURE COMPLEX CHANGE

While the search for a simple intervention technique has been fruitless, there has also been a vain search to find an easy test for the profound changes that result from psychotherapeutic intervention. In this attempt, it seems that we have confused clarity of thinking with narrowness of vision and have often resorted to what is measurable, rather than what is meaningful. Some researchers have limited themselves to overt behavior change as a criterion of psychotherapeutic effectiveness. But work with delinquents has taught us that this criterion is an extremely unreliable measure. For example, how does one quantify antisocial behaviors? Does an antisocial youth improve when he has gone from one assault-and-battery charge to three breaking-and-entering charges? In addition, in delinquency one is dealing with a problem within a social context. These young people have already been identified as antisocial in the community. Whenever community problems arise, these adolescents are the first to be accused whether or not they are indeed the culprits. Thus, they are labeled, provoked, and sometimes charged in ways that merely confirm the self-fulfilling prophecy.

Other researchers have spoken of personality change as the aim of psychotherapeutic intervention. But what personality change? How can we measure those changes objectively? As mentioned before, the broad question, Is psychotherapy effective?, was not asked in our study. Rather, the question was asked, What do we think should change in these antisocial youths as a result of psychotherapy, and how could this be measured? If necessary, for example, we would develop new measuring instruments. We concluded that change should be measured on three different levels: (1) overt behavior; (2) the area of cognition and learning (these youths, as mentioned before, were far behind in academic achievement, performing on the average at a third-grade level in reading, despite being in high school) ; and (3) personality structure change.

The overt behavioral level was handled descriptively. We took educational histories, job histories (including wages), legal histories, and other information about the general functioning of these youths.*

The cognitive area was measured by using standard achievement tests in reading, vocabulary, arithmetic fundamentals, and arithmetic problems. All these were administered individually.

To measure personality structure the question was asked, What specific personality areas did we expect to change? Three areas were selected for this antisocial group: self-image, control of aggression, and attitude toward authority. Note how the areas would not be appropriate for other pathological groups for whom one might have different treatment goals.

Pictures were selected in these three areas and the youths were asked to tell stories in the manner of the Thematic Apperception Test. These pictures had been selected by a group of psychologists for their stimulus relevance in eliciting responses related to self-image, control of aggression, and attitude toward authority. The young person's total response to the request to tell a story to the picture was evaluated. That is, the test situation was viewed as a task to be performed under certain standard stimulating conditions that would elicit patterns of ego functioning.

The tests were administered before treatment, immediately after treatment, and two years following treatment. Testing was done by a person other than the therapist. The material collected was then given to a third independent judge who was unfamiliar with the goals of the study, but was a highly experienced clinical psychologist. He was asked to judge these stories according to certain specifically

---

* An interesting finding was that marital status seemed associated with improvement. Those youths who improved, since they had some financial means, left home, married, and started families; those who did not improve remained single and, if they were not in jail or in a hospital, continued to live with their family of origin.

outlined criteria that had been derived from material obtained from sources other than these antisocial youths. The stories were randomized in such a way as to eliminate any possible biases and to obtain an objective measure of whether there was any change resulting from treatment.

To test the effectiveness of the program, 20 youths who met the criteria were randomly assigned to two groups, one treated by our comprehensive vocationally oriented psychotherapy, and one left to the resources available in the community. Analysis revealed that these groups were identical at the start of the program.

The results, after 10 months of treatment, showed significant changes in all areas in the treated group when compared to the untreated group (Massimo and Shore, 1963). In overt behavior there was a noticeable decline in legal problems in the treated young people. Job performance improved and wages rose. Most of the youths decided to undertake some sort of education program, either by returning to public school or through alternative academic channels. Despite the difficulties in learning they had had for many years, the young people treated by comprehensive vocationally oriented psychotherapy showed a significant improvement in all areas of achievement—reading, vocabulary, arithmetic fundamentals and arithmetic problems. With respect to personality functioning, significant changes were found in self-image and control of aggression. Attitudes toward authority did change, but the changes were not significant. This finding seemed consistent with some of the struggles for independence expected in adolescence, with opposition to authority common among well-adjusted as well as antisocial adolescent youth.

IV. DOES CHANGE WASH OUT OVER TIME?

Unfortunately, there are few follow-up studies in our field that could help us understand not only the nature of change but the relationship of change to later development. It has become typical for us to think in terms of immediate visible results, not looking beyond the short life of a program. However, we were interested in and were able to study what happened to our youths after treatment ended. These young people were retested with all the tests two years after the program ended (Shore and Massimo, 1966). Five and ten years after treatment, they were interviewed to determine their functioning (Shore and Massimo, 1969, 1973). The results showed that not only did they continue to change (although the pace of improvement seemed to slow down after treatment), but other events occurred in their lives. For example, one major finding was that, over the 10-year period, not one young person reversed direction. Thus, if the adolescent youth improved over the 10-month period when he was 15 to 17 years old, he did well when he was 25 to 27 years old. Those who showed a drop over that 10-month period continued to decline. None of the youths who had experience with either state hospitals or jails, that is, with institutions set up to supposedly rehabilitate people, was able to reverse this direction.

V. So WHAT DOES THIS TELL US ABOUT PEOPLE?

One of the major sources of dissension between the field of program evaluation and that of research has been the question of what the data tell us about the nature of change and of personality functioning. Program evaluation often has been seen as a way of determining whether or not a particular program works and should continue. Why certain interventions work while others do not work is a question seldom asked. Program evaluators have been criticized for not attempting to look at what happens in treatment. I believe that program evaluation, without an effort to study the phenomenon being evaluated, merely becomes a management tool for manipulating staff, securing funds, or selling a program for reasons other than its contribution to our knowledge and understanding of people. True, our first concern in this project was, Did this program work? But the evaluation was organized in such a way as to explore why and how it might have worked. For that reason we analyzed and reanalyzed our data and collected more material on a second control group.

Since we had a large number of stories, achievement tests, and descriptive data on the treated and untreated groups, we were able to undertake a variety of new analyses to determine the nature of change.

The second control group from which we collected more data was a group of nondelinquent adolescent youths matched by age and socioeconomic level to the youths in the program. These nondelinquent youths were tested in the same manner as those in the program over a 10-month period to determine the changes that might take place as a result of normal changes in adolescence. Some of our findings shed light on the nature of delinquency in adolescent young people, as well as on the nature of change in psychotherapy.

Special scales were developed to analyze different aspects of ego-functioning on the stories to the pictures: guilt (Shore, Massimo, and Mack, 1964; Shore et al., 1968a), object relations (Shore et al., 1966, 1968b), perception of role functioning (Shore, Massimo, and Mack, 1965), concept of time—future and past (Ricks, Umbarger, and Mack, 1964), and verbalization (Shore and Massimo, 1967). All were analyzed on the stories given before, immediately after, and two years after treatment for the three groups—the treated group, the untreated group, and the nondelinquent group. Some of our findings are of interest. On the concept of time, treated delinquents showed a significantly greater increase in orientation toward the future than did the untreated delinquents. Neither the treated nor the untreated delinquent youths showed any change in their view of the past. Adolescence, it appears, is a time for looking forward rather than back.

Verbalization showed a significant increase in areas related to aggressive stimulation (Shore, Massimo, and Moran, 1967). Therefore, verbalization seems to be one mechanism by which control over antisocial behavior can be developed. The use of words in successfully treated adolescent delinquent youths was greater under the stimuli that elicited aggressive content than even that displayed by the nondelinquent youth.

The learning problems in the adolescent delinquent youths were found to be related to the socialization process and the rejection of learning as part of socialization, rather than to the neurotic interactions which have been described in many cases of adolescent learning problems (Shore et al., 1966). Once this resistance to socialization was dealt with, there was significant improvement in all areas of academic learning—reading, vocabulary, arithmetic fundamentals and arithmetic problems (Shore, Massimo, and Ricks, 1965). The successful change in these antisocial youths seemed related to redirecting of their high energy levels into more socialized channels, rather than in reducing their activity. One is led to believe that there may even be a constitutional basis for the high energy level of these youths.

Our chronic delinquent adolescents also seemed to be qualitatively different from nondelinquents in their ways of dealing with the world (Shore, Massimo, and Moran, 1967). Cognitively, for example, the antisocial youths were more aware of people and seemed more attuned to interactions between people in a way that indicated heightened ego-functioning in areas relevant to manipulation of the environment and people. It seemed that part of the ego structure of antisocial youths might be an increased sensitivity to opportunities for manipulation and self-gratification, something clinicians have observed and that has been so vividly described by Redl and Wineman (1957). These are only some of our findings.

Let me conclude by noting some important national trends. There is a growing concern with service and service-delivery issues, particularly services to children and youth. This concern should increase as the United States begins to develop a national policy toward children and youth similar to that of many European nations. With this increase in concern, however, will come an even greater interest in accountability. What do we do? How do we do it? What effect does it have? How do we know? How much does it cost? As a result, we have had a proliferation of management techniques—management by objectives, goal-attainment scaling, and other ways of evaluating mental health programs. In fact, evaluation has now become a major part of programming for any mental health service if it is to obtain any public funding. This emphasis on evaluation means that therapeutic-intervention research is now of more than academic interest. It is essential that we develop ways of evaluating and studying the effectiveness of our interventions—ways that lead to knowledge about ourselves as well as satisfying those interested in such issues as management and cost-effectiveness. With an anticipated increase in funding, new programs and new opportunities will arise for creative work on therapeutic change. It is through our ingenuity that we will be able to use this current concern with program evaluation to develop the knowledge that can form the basis for planning intelligent and meaningful social policy. We hoped by undertaking this project to contribute to that goal in some way.

REFERENCES

BERGIN, A. E., and GARFIELD, S. L. (eds.). 1971. *Handbook of Psychotherapy and Behavior Change.* New York: Wiley.

BERGIN, A. E. and STRUPP, H. H. 1972. *Changing Frontiers in the Science of Psychotherapy.* Chicago: Aldine.

EYSENCK, H. J. 1952. The effects of psychotherapy. *J. Consult. Psychol.,* 16:319-324.

HEINICKE, C. M., and STRASSMANN, L. H. 1975. Toward more effective research in child psychotherapy. *J. Am. Acad. Child Psychiatry,* 14 (4):561-588.

MASSIMO, J. L., and SHORE, M. F. 1963. The effectiveness of a vocationally oriented psychotherapy program for adolescent delinquent boys. *Am. J. Orthopsychiatry,* 33:634-643.

MASSIMO, J. L., and SHORE, M. F. 1967. Comprehensive vocationally oriented psychotherapy: A new treatment technique for lower class adolescent delinquent youth. *Psychiatry,* 30:229-236.

MELTZOFF, J., and KORNREICH, M. 1970. *Research in Psychotherapy.* New York: Atherton Press.

REDL, F., and WINEMAN, D. 1957. *The Aggressive Child.* New York: Free Press (Macmillan).

RICKS, D., UMBARGER, C., and MACK, R. 1964. A measure of increased temporal perspective in successfully treated adolescent delinquent boys. *J. Abnorm. Soc. Psychol.,* 69:685-689.

SHORE, M. F., and MASSIMO, J. L. 1966. Comprehensive vocationally oriented psychotherapy for adolescent delinquent boys: A follow-up study. *Am. J. Orthopsychiatry,* 36:609-616.

SHORE, M. F., and MASSIMO, J. L. 1967. Verbalization, stimulus relevance, and personality change. *J. Consult. Psychol.* 31:423-424.

SHORE, M. F., and MASSIMO, J. L. 1969. Five years later: A follow-up study of comprehensive, vocationally oriented psychotherapy. *Am. J. Orthopsychiatry,* 39 (5): 769-774.

SHORE, M. F., and MASSIMO, J. L. 1973. After ten years: A follow-up study of comprehensive, vocationally oriented psychotherapy. *Am. J. Orthopsychiatry,* 43 (1): 128-132.

SHORE, M. F., MASSIMO, J. L., KISIELEWSKI, J., and MORAN, J. K. 1966. Object relations changes resulting from successful psychotherapy with adolescent delinquents and their relationship to academic performance. *J. Am. Acad. Child Psychiatry,* 5:93-104.

SHORE, M. F., MASSIMO, J. L., and MACK, R. 1964. The relationship between levels of guilt in thematic stories and unsocialized behavior. *Journal of Projective Techniques and Personality Assessment,* 28:346-349.

SHORE, M. F., MASSIMO, J. L., and MACK, R. 1965. Changes in the perception of interpersonal relations in successfully treated adolescent delinquent boys. *J. Consult. Psychol.,* 29:213-217.

SHORE, M. F., MASSIMO, J. L., MACK, R., and MALASKY, C. 1968a. Studies of psychotherapeutic change in adolescent delinquent boys: The role of guilt. *Psychotherapy,* 5:85-89.

SHORE, M. F., MASSIMO, J. L., and MORAN, J. K. 1967. Some cognitive dimensions of interpersonal behavior in adolescent delinquent boys. *Journal of Research in Crime and Delinquency,* 4:243-248.

SHORE, M. F., MASSIMO, J. L., MORAN, J. K., and MALASKY, C. 1968b. Object relations changes and psychotherapeutic intervention: A follow-up study. *J. Am. Acad. Child Psychiatry,* 7:59-68.

SHORE, M. F., MASSIMO, J. L., and RICKS, D. F. 1965. A factor analytic study of psychotherapeutic change in delinquent boys. *J. Clin. Psychol.,* 21:208-212.

8

Psychopharmacotherapy in Children

ROBERT L. SPRAGUE, Ph.D.

Psychopharmacotherapy in children has received wide public attention in the 1970s and has generated a number of basic questions. This paper is concerned with the fundamental questions being raised about psychotropic drug treatment of children by parents, by teachers, by researchers, and, last but certainly not least, the public media.

Although the public interest in drug treatment for children waxes and wanes, it has remained at a high level since the Omaha incident in which it was reported by television news commentators that a large percentage, perhaps 20 to 25 percent, of children in the Omaha School District were receiving stimulant medication for hyperactivity. This story was later circulated in print (Maynard, 1970) and subsequently proven to be substantially in error, especially the statements about prevalence of drug usage.

The prevalence of drug usage is the first basic question and will be addressed in this paper. From the time of the news release there has been continued interest in the use of psychotropic drugs for the treatment of hyperactive or MBD (minimally brain-dysfunctioned) children. In fact, two free-lance authors (Schrag and Divoky, 1975) have written a popular book with the main theme that hyperactivity is a myth created and propounded by a conspiracy of doctors,

The preparation of this paper was supported in part by PHS Research Grant No. MH 18909 from the National Institute of Mental Health and Grant No. HD 05951 from the National Institute of Child Health and Human Development.

teachers, school administrators, and parents—a most unlikely collection of conspirators in view of the fact that these co-conspirators cannot agree on anything else such as taxes for teachers' salaries. These authors are very concerned about the effects of psychotropic drugs on school performance of the child; this is the second basic question to be addressed in this paper. An active interest in this topic is also demonstrated by professionals, as evidenced by the almost 1900 publications on the topic (Winchell, 1975) and the recent publication of two comprehensive textbooks (Ross and Ross, 1976; Safer and Allen, 1976).

All of the previous comments concerned hyperactivity and drug treatment in children. Similar interest and controversy are rapidly brewing about drug treatment of the mentally retarded (Mosher, 1975). It has been claimed in the popular press that there is extensive overuse of psychotropic medication with the mentally retarded and a number of lawsuits have been filed in the federal courts with this as an issue. Thus, the third basic question is the public impact of these controversies.

I have outlined the basic plan of this paper in which I will discuss three basic issues arising from pharmacotherapy in children. These basic issues will be discussed with reference to two populations of children—the hyperactive and the mentally retarded.

PREVALENCE OF DRUG THERAPY

Mentally Retarded

Although most of the stories about high frequency of psychotropic drug treatment for children relate to the hyperactive child, factual information about prevalence of drug treatment first came from the mentally retarded population. Dr. Ronald S. Lipman of the Psychopharmacology Research Branch of the National Institute of Mental Health conducted the first study of prevalence of psychotropic drug treatment in 1966-67 and reported on the use of psychotropic drugs with institutionalized mentally retarded residents (Lipman, 1970). He mailed questionnaires about the use of psychotropic drugs to all residential institutions for the mentally retarded in the United States.

The following data were reported: (1) 51 percent of the residents were receiving psychotropic drugs; (2) two major tranquilizers, thioridazine and chlorpromazine, accounted for 58 percent of all reported psychotropic drugs, with maximum dosage much above manufacturer's recommendations; (3) 22 percent of the residents typically received these medications for four or more years.

About nine years after this initial survey, DiMascio (1975) reported on the use of psychotropic drugs in two institutions in Massachusetts, one facility housing 2132 patients and the other housing 878 patients. In the large facility 26 percent of the patients were receiving psychotropic drugs whereas 53 percent of the patients were receiving psychotropic drugs in the smaller facility where the more severely impaired patients were located.

In 1976 we completed two surveys of the use of psychotropic drugs in the *total* population of two institutions in the midwest (Sprague, 1976b) ; one was a large, old institution housing 1638 patients, the other a new, small institution with 286 patients. The mean age of patients of both institutions was about 28 years; the mean length of time in the large facility was about 17 years whereas it was only one year in the small institution that had recently opened. In the large institution 67.2 percent and in the small institution 65.4 percent of the patients were receiving psychotropic and anticonvulsant drugs. Although there are many differences between the two facilities in terms of size, ratio of staff to patients, and, most important, philosophy of the institution, the rank order of type of drug used is about the same for both institutions. The order of usage of the three most popular drugs is identical: (1) thioridazine, (2) diphenylhydantoin, and (3) phenobarbital.

In general, the mean dosages are relatively high for most of the drugs and the ranges, particularly the upper end of the dosage range, are extremely high for the large institution. Lipman found that about 22 percent of the patients were receiving psychotropic drugs indefinitely, that is, the patients were on medication for an indefinite or a very long period of time. Fortunately, the tendency for very long prescription periods seems to have changed in the last 10 years, as indicated by our survey. In the large institution, thioridazine had been given for an average of almost three years, diphenylhydantoin for an average of about four years, phenobarbital for somewhat more than three years, chlorpromazine for about two years, and diazepam for about two years.

Hyperactive Children

The first national estimate of the prevalence of drug therapy for hyperactivity was given by Lipman before a Congressional subcommittee (Gallagher, 1970). He speculated that between 150,000 and 200,000 children were receiving medication for hyperactivity. One of our colleagues, Karen Stephen (Sprague and Sleator, 1973), sent a questionnaire to about 700 physicians in the greater metropolitan Chicago area. From the returned questionnaires she estimated the number of children who had received psychotropic drugs. Comparing this figure to the total number of children enrolled in the Chicago schools, she speculated that between 2 and 4 percent of the elementary school children had received drug therapy for hyperactivity during the 1970-71 school year. Stimulants were the most frequently prescribed drugs with the average duration of therapy being nine months. Dosage information obtained from the Stephen study indicated an average dose from 6.5 mg/day for dextroamphetamine for children under five years of age, to 14 mg/day for adolescents; corresponding figures for methylphenidate are 11.5 mg and 24.5 mg. As we have pointed out before, these dosages prescribed by practicing physicians are well below those typically recommended by some authorities (Sprague and Sleator, 1973, 1975, 1976). The most comprehensive data available about the prevalence of drug therapy for hyperactivity were reported by Krager and Safer (1974) in surveys of school nurses conducted in 1971 and again in 1973 in Baltimore County, Maryland. The authors report that in 1973, 1.73 percent of the 66,000 school children were receiving drugs for hyperactivity. This prevalence (1.73 percent) was a 62 percent increase over the prevalence reported in the survey conducted in 1971 (1.07 percent). Stimulants accounted for 88.2 percent of all therapeutic drugs, with methylphenidate the most common. In sharp contrast to what is reported in the media, the prevalence was greater for school districts with above-mean income (1.81 percent) in comparison to the prevalence in districts with below-mean income (1.64 percent). Thus, there are no empirical data to support the many sensational stories to the effect that economically disadvantaged people are singled out by physicians for excessively high prescription rates of psychotropic drugs.

A more recent estimate was given by Scoville (1974) who used data from the 1973 National Diseases and Therapeutic Index and the National Prescription Audit. For children under the age of 10, 493,000 prescriptions were written for methylphenidate and 178,000 prescriptions for amphetamines—a total of 671,000 prescriptions for stimulants. Assuming that few prescriptions for hyperactivity were written for children over 10 and, again, assuming that the average prescription is for 30 days, Scoville estimated that the 671,000 prescriptions would account for treating 225,000 children for three months or 56,000 children for a full year. But it must be pointed out that both assumptions are questionable considering the nature of data collected by both indices (Sprague and Gadow, 1976).

A student (Gadow, 1975) surveyed all teachers in early-childhood special education programs in Illinois with the exception of Chicago. These programs serve three- to five-year-old children with learning problems, developmental delays, and handicaps ranging from mild to severe. His first survey of the 2000 children in these programs found that 12.6 percent received psychotropic or anticonvulsant drugs some time during the 1973-74 school year. Methylphenidate, diphenyl-hydantoin, and phenobarbital accounted for 62 percent of all reported drugs. In a survey the following year, 1974-75, Gadow (1976) found a slight increase in the prevalence of the usage of psychotropic and anticonvulsant drugs to 14 percent of the children. Of about 2500 children in the survey, 8 percent received medication for hyperactivity sometime during the school year. Stimulants accounted for 63 percent of all drugs reportedly used for hyperactivity.

Taking these reported facts and using census figures, we (Sprague and Gadow, 1976) have recently attempted to *estimate* the prevalence of psychotropic drug usage among school children in this country. If one uses the 2 percent figure obtained from Stephen's study (Sprague and Sleator, 1973) for the base population of children from kindergarten through eighth grade (34,400,000 for the fall of 1974), one obtains a figure of 688,000 children receiving psychotropic drugs. However, if one applies the same 2 percent prevalence to the base population of pupils from kindergarten through high school (50,010,000 for the fall of 1974), one obtains a figure of 1,000,200. Probably the best estimate is to use the Krager and Safer (1974) prevalence figure of 1.73 percent and the base population of children from kindergarten through eighth grade; these figures give an estimate of 595,120 children. But I want to reiterate that these are estimates with considerable error. What we are doing is taking the sampling estimate of the percentage of children on psychotropic drugs and multiplying sampling estimate by census data. This mean that a very small sampling error in percentage of prevalence leads to very large errors in absolute numbers of children estimated to be on psychotropic medication; for example, an error of only 0.01 percent in the percentage estimate leads to a difference of 5,000 children in the estimate of the number of children receiving such medication.

Summarizing the prevalence data, the percentage of school-age children receiving psychotropic medication in the United States is certainly much lower than the alarming percentages reported in the public press. Nevertheless, the numbers of such children are substantial—about 500,000 to 600,000. For the population of institutionalized mentally retarded, the picture is entirely different. The prevalence rate is probably 60 to 65 percent. An estimate of the institutionalized retarded population in the United States is about 200,000 which, with an incidence of 60 percent, would lead to 120,000 individuals on psychotropic drugs.

Effects on School Performance

Social Behavior

Hyperactivity. In this paper the term "social behavior" will be used to refer to the behavior of the child under study, usually the

CONNERS' ABBREVIATED TEACHER RATING SCALE

CHILD'S NAME _____   CODE NUMBER _____
                                         STUDY NUMBER _____

TEACHER'S OBSERVATIONS
    Information obtained _____ by _____
                         month   day   year

Observation	Degree of Activity			
	Not at all	Just a little	Pretty much	Very much
1. Restless and overactive				
2. Excitable, impulsive				
3. Disturbs other children				
4. Fails to finish things he starts – short attention span				
5. Constantly fidgeting				
6. Inattentive, easily distracted				
7. Demands must be met immediately – easily frustrated				
8. Cries easily and often				
9. Mood changes quickly and drastically				
10. Temper outbursts, explosive and unpredictable behavior				

OTHER OBSERVATIONS OF TEACHER

FIGURE 1. Conners' Abbreviated Teacher Rating Scale.

hyperactive child, in the classroom situation as perceived by a significant adult, primarily the teacher. The most widely used teacher-evaluation procedure is the Conners' Teacher Rating Scale (Conners, 1969), a four-point scale with 39 items. The scale was subsequently shortened to 10 items (Conners, et al., 1972) (Figure 1).

There are three main advantages of the Conners' scale: (1) it has been used repeatedly and successfully in drug studies (Sprague and Werry, 1974); (2) normative data have been obtained; and (3) it has been analyzed into factors that can be replicated (Werry, Sprague, and Cohen, 1975). In a study of 178 children in New York City, normative data were obtained in a study which manipulated psychotropic drugs and placebo (Kupietz, Bialer, and Winsberg, 1972). In one of our studies normative data were obtained for 291 normal classmate cohorts of a group of 64 hyperactive children on the Conners' scale (Sprague, Christensen, and Werry, 1974). From these data it is clear that teachers can distinguish the hyperactive child from the normal child in their classrooms and, further, that a score of 15 on the Abbreviated Conners' Rating Scale, of a possible total score of 30, would place the child in the upper 2.5 percent of the distribution of children rated with the scale. This upper 2.5 percent is a convenient statistical cutoff which is two standard deviations above the mean for the normal sample. The cutoff of 15 is now being widely accepted as a standard diagnostic procedure in evaluating hyperactive children, at least in research studies.

Another technique that has been used to obtain quantitative information about the behavior of a child in the classroom is systematic observation by an adult not identified with the school system. Such an observation technique has been described by Werry and Quay (1969).

When one of these two techniques, the rating scale or an independent observer is used, the effects of stimulant drugs on the social behavior of hyperactive children are easily detected. About three years ago we reviewed all the studies on the effects of psychotropic drugs on social behavior in school (Sprague and Werry, 1974). We discovered that *every* time the Conners' Rating Scale had been used, statistically significant results had been obtained indicating that teacher ratings showed improvement when stimulant medications were used with hyperactive children in comparison to a placebo condition. When the child was receiving stimulants, the teachers typically perceived the hyperactive child as more attentive, less socially aggressive, less disruptive, less impulsive, less active, and having fewer temper outbursts.

In the current climate of controversy about psychotropic drug treatment of hyperactive children, the critics would certainly argue that one cannot trust teacher ratings because, as the critics would state it, the teachers are part of a repressive school system that forces enthusiastic, effervescent children into rigid molds for benefit of a capitalistic society. The independent-observer technique avoids this criticism because the observer records as directly as possible the actual behavior of the child in the class. When the observation technique is used, generally the same results are found, namely that the administration of stimulant medication to hyperactive children results in better social behavior in the classroom (Sprague, Barnes, and Werry, 1970).

A word of caution should be issued, however, about making final decisions from only one domain of behavior, that is, social behavior. As we have pointed out (Sprague and Sleator, 1973, 1975), there is evidence that the dosage of stimulant medication required to produce the greatest improvement in social behavior leads to an actual reduction in learning performance.

At this point let us turn to the second important aspect of school performance, namely learning performance.

Learning Performance

Background. Psychopharmacology (Russell, 1960), particularly pediatric psychopharmacology (DiMascio, 1970; Sprague and Sleator, 1975) has been criticized for its overdependence on empiricism with a lack of theory. One possible interface between behavior theory and pediatric psychopharmacology is in the area of learning of the child. A large body of literature exists regarding the learning of the child; several theories have been developed, for example, to explain differences observed between the learning performance of retarded and normal children (Zeaman and House, 1963; Ellis, 1970) .

Following the leads of theorists like Zeaman and House, we (Sprague and Sleator, 1975, 1976) used a picture-recognition task (Scott, 1971) of short-term memory to monitor the effects of psychotropic drugs on learning performance. The task involves showing the child one or several pictures of common objects for a few seconds, turning the picture off, and then, a few seconds later, presenting a single test picture to which the child is to respond. The child's task is to indicate whether he saw the test picture in the previous presentation by pressing a lever labeled "same" which indicates he saw it before, or a lever labeled "different" which indicates he did not see it. Obviously, a child cannot perform successfully on this task unless he pays attention to the picture presentation and has a good memory during the four-second interval. The initial display usually consists of three, nine, or 15 common pictures, a brief blank interval of four seconds, and then the test probe which is left on the screen until the child responds to it by pressing one of the levers.

A number of features of this task make it especially useful in studying drug effects on learning: (1) it is sensitive to information load, that is, the greater the number of stimuli (pictures) in the initial presentation matrix, the lower the accuracy on the test trial, which allows the experimenter to set appropriate levels of accuracy for children who vary widely in intellectual ability; (2) after initial pretraining in a few sessions, accuracy of performance reaches a plateau, and there is little subsequent change over many experimental sessions, which makes this an ideal test to be used repeatedly; (3) relatively little change in performance occurs within one experimental session; (4) the accuracy and the latency of responding seem to represent two independent measures of performance on the task as work by Scott (1971) clearly indicates; (5) most important, children like the game.

In a long series of studies investigating the effects of psychotropic drugs on both social behavior and learning performance of hyperactive children, we typically use a within-subject or crossover design. In such a crossover design, every child participates in every dosage or drug condition. Usually each drug or dosage condition will last for three or four weeks. The child is brought to the laboratory at the end of each dosage period and tested on the learning task. Information is also obtained, usually at weekly intervals, from the teacher about the child's performance in the classroom.

After extensive evaluations are completed and the child is accepted into one of our studies, and the parents have signed written consent forms, close contact is maintained with the family during the duration of the experiment, usually three or four months. Three or four dosage conditions are typically used. The child's regular teacher completes the Conners' Abbreviated Rating Scale weekly. At the end of each dosage condition, the parent fills out the same scale, brings the child back to the laboratory for testing, for examination by the pediatrician, for interviews by the social worker, and for prescription refills. Great care is taken to ensure that the child receives the medication as prescribed. All medication is dispensed in orange opaque capsules that conceal the tablets from sight and taste. For a particular child, each capsule always contains the same number of tablets; the number of placebo tablets varies according to the dosage under study. Each parent is given a file box with a supply of medicine in individual, dated envelopes. Parents are told that forgetting to open an envelope and giving a capsule to the child is not a catastrophe, and they are instructed to return unopened envelopes so that missed days can be recorded. Each parent usually returns a few unopened envelopes. Medication is always given in the morning before school by one parent.

Strict double-blind procedures are used. Only one member of the investigative team, a person who does not have direct contact with the child, knows the drug-sequence code. The pediatrician can obtain this information from that team member any time an emergency arises. It has been our experience that the few times a code has been broken by the pediatrician for what seemed an emergency, the child was on placebo more often than on drug.

Hyperactive children. Taking data from both the domain of social behavior and learning performance and plotting these data against

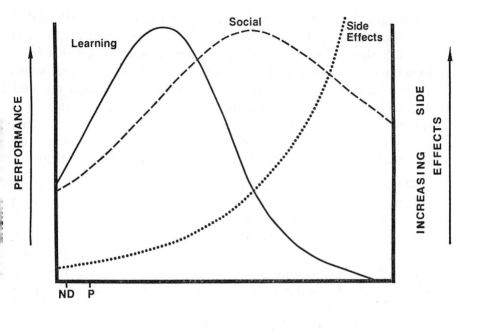

FIGURE 2. Theoretical dose-response curves for stimulants with
hyperactive children. *ND*—no drug, *P*—placebo.

dosages on a mg/kg basis, we have consistently obtained two different
dose-response curves (Sprague and Sleator, 1976). For hyperactive
children, there is always a statistically significant enhancement of
learning performance on the picture recognition task as one moves
from placebo to a low-dosage condition until a peak enhancement
is reached at 0.3 mg/kg, beyond which increases in dosage lead to a
decline in learning performance. This is one dose-response curve.
For social behavior, there is continued improvement in teacher ratings from placebo to low dosages until a peak enhancement is reached
about 1.0 mg/kg. This is the other dose-response curve (Figure 2).

The intriguing aspect of these two dose-response curves is that the
peak improvement in learning performance and social behavior does
not occur at the same dosage level. Thus, if one wants to enhance

learning, a dosage of 0.3 mg/kg (which is about one-seventh of that recommended as optimal by the authoritative Goodman and Gilman [1970]), should be prescribed. If one prescribes a dosage that leads to maximum improvement of social behavior in the classroom, about 1.0 mg/kg, performance on the learning task declines below the level of placebo. These data are important, we believe, because they indicate to the physician that the target behavior for which the medicine is prescribed should be carefully selected and monitored because not all behaviors of the child respond equally to variations in dosage.

Mentally retarded children. Unfortunately from a number of viewpoints, the data and theory about the effects of psychotropic drugs on the learning performance of the mentally retarded child are much less complete than the above description of the hyperactive child. In an earlier paper on methodology (Sprague and Werry, 1971), we surveyed all psychotropic drug studies available in the literature which involved the mentally retarded—182 studies, of which only seven used some kind of learning measure. We recently reviewed the results of these studies (Sprague and Werry, 1974) and I will simply quote from the summary of the mentally retarded section of that paper.

> . . . there are very few studies from the vast literature on the psychopharmacology of the MR [mentally retarded] that address themselves to educational issues, issues such as learning performance, gains in achievement, or social behavior in the classroom. In the studies reviewed, it seems quite clear that the tranquilizing drugs led to reduction in stereotyped movements. However, the unanswered question is whether this reduction in stereotypy was obtained at a loss in alertness and ability to learn new tasks. The studies using the stimulants present a mixed picture. Probably the best interpretation is that the stimulants would influence the MR in the same way that they affect hyperactive or MBD [minimal brain dysfunction] children. However, a good test of this particular hypothesis remains to be performed. What is clear is that psychotropic drugs are used heavily. It is equally apparent that the main problem of the MR is slow learning and that their behavioral problems are all too often handled by administering large amounts of tranquilizing drugs which characteristically suppress learning. Thus, for treatment, the MR

are often placed in institutions where social stimulation is reduced, where tranquilizing drugs which suppress learning are
administered in large amounts, and where, ironically, it is expected that these combinations should produce new skills to
enable the retarded to become rehabilitated members of the
community.

IMPACT ON THE PUBLIC

Food and Drug Administration

The Food and Drug Administration (FDA) is legally charged with
the task of certifying any drugs that are approved for interstate marketing, closely monitoring the research of pharmaceutical firms as
they prepare new drugs for possible marketing, and surveillance of
the marketing and advertising practices of firms after the drugs are
certified. The FDA has been under close scrutiny and considerable
criticism over recent years (Silverman and Lee, 1974). Much of the
criticism of the agency has been aimed at the way the FDA has
monitored the research and marketing practices of pharmaceutical
firms. Major changes have been made in the FDA in the last few
years. In my opinion, one of the most notable changes was the ap-
pointment of a variety of scientific advisory bodies to review research
of drug firms and advise the agency on scientific merit of the research.
The outside consultants, "experts" as they are called by the FDA,
have opened the entire review process to public scrutiny and have
provided a more capable review in the sense that the FDA now has
a large number of specialists available as needed rather than a more
limited number of specialists employed as scientists by the agency.

In July 1974, the FDA appointed a committee of 11 specialists to
form the Pediatric Advisory Subcommittee to review psychotropic
drugs used with children in the United States.* One of the first tasks

---

* The members of the subcommittee are: Bonnie W. Camp, University of Colorado
Medical Center, pediatrician and psychologist; C. Keith Conners, University of Pitts-
burg Medical School, pediatric psychopharmacologist; Rachel Gittelman, Hillside Hospital, psychopharmacologist; Ronald S. Lipman, National Institute of Mental Health,
psychopharmacologist; Robert Moore, University of California at San Diego, pediatric
neurologist; Judith L. Rapaport, National Institute of Mental Health, child psychiatrist; Robert Reichler, University of Washington, child psychiatrist; Lee N.
Robins, Washington School of Medicine, Sociologist; Donald Robinson, University of
Vermont, pharmacologist; Gabrielle C. Weiss, Montreal Children's Hospital, child
psychiatrist; and I am chairman and claim to be a pediatric psychopharmacologist.

assigned to the subcommittee was to review the use of psychotropic drugs with the institutionalized retarded in the United States. The issue was brought to the subcommittee in a petition filed by the Washington law firm of Hogan and Hartson. After several meetings with the lawyers of this firm and outside consultants and a review of the large literature on this question, the advisory group issued a report to the agency. The essential points of this report were made public in a letter by then Commissioner Schmidt to the law firm.

The petitioners had asked for seven specific actions by the FDA, and the commissioner approved several of these requests. The actions the commissioner approved are: revised labeling of some of the phenothiazines, revised labeling of some drugs to clearly specify the behavior problems for which they should be administered, labeling to include precautions about monitoring the effects with the retarded who have difficulty in verbal communication, and a promise that warnings and precautions about the use of psychotropic drugs would be issued from time to time when necessary.

A series of lawsuits has been filed involving the use of psychotropic drugs with the mentally retarded. A brief accounting of the most important lawsuits follows. In the landmark case of *Wyatt* v. *Stickney* (The *Wyatt* case, 1975) a group of consumer, legal, and professional organizations filed a lawsuit on behalf of a patient at Partlow State School in Tuscaloosa, Alabama, for legal relief of understaffing, underfinancing, overcrowding, and poor medical care in a large state institution for the retarded. Judge Frank M. Johnson ordered a number of changes which were upheld on appeal to the appellate court (*Wyatt* v. *Anderholt,* 1974). In a section of his order entitled medication, Judge Johnson ordered the following changes: (1) no medication shall be administered unless it is on the written order of a physician; (2) records of the medication prescribed and weekly review by the physician were also ordered—prescriptions were not to exceed 30 days; (3) "residents will have the right to be free from unnecessary or excessive medication"; (4) "medication shall not be used as punishment, for the convenience of staff, as a substitute for a habilitative program, or in quantities that interfere with the resident's habilitative period"; and (5) pharmacy services to be directed by competent, professionally trained pharmacists were ordered.

In another major case, *New York State Association for Retarded Children* v. *Nelson Rockefeller* (1975), a consent decree (that is, both plaintiff and defendant agreed on terms of a settlement) ordered 23 sets of standards ranging from community placement to medication to speech and audiology services. Appendix Q, medication, includes the orders issued in the Wyatt case plus the following orders: (1) "Notation of each individual's medication shall be kept in his medical records. At least weekly the attending physician shall review the drug regimen of each resident under his care." (2) "The resident's record shall state the effects of psychoactive medication on the resident. When dosages of psychoactive medication are changed or other psychoactive medications are prescribed, a notation shall be made in the resident's record concerning the effect of the new medication or new dosages and the behavior changes, if any, which occur." (3) "Only appropriately trained staff shall be allowed to administer drugs." (4) "Written policies and procedures that govern the safe administration and handling of all drugs shall be developed." (5) "Drugs shall be stored under proper conditions." (6) "Discontinued and outdated drugs . . . shall be returned to the pharmacy for proper disposition." (7) "Medication errors and drug reactions shall be recorded and reported immediately to the practitioner who ordered the drug."

These previous cases involve suits against public institutions. A loophole has existed in the sense that many retarded people are placed in privately operated facilities in the community that are subsidized by state and/or federal funds but are not under the direct regulation of the federal government. Often retarded children in these facilities are from other states. A few years ago in my home state of Illinois, a controversy erupted about the Illinois Department of Children and Family Services' placing more than 500 foster children in facilities in Texas where the parents found it difficult or impossible to visit (Sprague, 1976a).

In what will probably be another landmark case (*Gary W.* v. *State of Louisiana,* 1976), an attorney filed on behalf of a Louisiana adolescent placed in a Texas private facility a suit against the State of Louisiana and private facilities in Texas. The attorney was soon joined by consumer legal groups and by the Office of Special Litigation of the U.S. Department of Justice (Velie, 1976). During site visits to some of the private facilities for the Office of Special Litigation, I found deplorable conditions involving extensive use of psychotropic medication, often for long periods of time at high doses. For example, in one facility for severely retarded children, the average stay for patients was 7.8 years with 66 percent of the patients regularly receiving anticonvulsant medication. The physician supervising these patients had ordered only one laboratory test to monitor this medication in 184.3 patient-years (a patient-year is one patient in that facility one year). Judge Alvin B. Rubin, who sifted through 47,000 pages of exhibits plus 3300 pages of depositions developed by 18 lawyers, has issued a preliminary decision in the case. It seems likely that the standards established in the two cases mentioned above will be followed in this case.

Hyperactive Children

The first lawsuit involving the use of stimulants with hyperactive children who are attending public schools has been filed in California—*Benskin* v. *Taft City School District* (Bruck, 1976). The suit was filed by the Youth Law Center of San Francisco on behalf of several parents of children who were receiving methylphenidate. Because there has not been a hearing on this litigation, the outcome is not known at this time. However, whatever the outcome, the results will certainly be of interest to many people.

SUMMARY

The issue of psychopharmacotherapy of children has caught the public eye. Publicity about drug treatment of children for behavioral problems has created public controversy. Three basic questions generated by this controversy were discussed in this paper. Although a low percentage of school children are receiving psychotropic medication, less than 2 percent, the absolute number of children in the

United States is large, possibly 500,000 to 600,000. On the other hand, although the population of institutionalized mentally retarded children is small, the percentage of these patients receiving psychotropic drugs is large and growing, about 60 percent.

What are the effects of psychotropic drugs on children's school performance? For the stimulant drugs for hyperactive children, the evidence is quite clear that the medication improves social behavior and at low doses leads to enhanced learning performance. On the other hand, neuroleptic medication for the institutionalized retarded reduces bizarre and stereotyped behavior apparently at the expense of suppressing learning performance.

This controversy and publicity have had an impact. The FDA has responded to the challenge and issued a number of warnings and has relabeled medication. Further changes in regulations are likely. A series of lawsuits is underway, particularly concerning the institutionalized child, forcing rapid upgrading of the standards for psychopharmacotherapy.

In summary, I urge physicians practicing psychopharmacotherapy with children to diagnose their patients carefully, to prescribe drugs conservatively and at conservative doses, and to monitor carefully and record the behavioral effects of these medications. If the medical community does not rapidly increase the quality of psychopharmacotherapy of children, the courts most assuredly will impose standards for that care.

REFERENCES

Bruck, C. 1976. Battle lines in the Ritalin war. *Human Behavior,* August, pp. 23-33.

Conners, C. K. 1969. A teacher rating scale for use in drug studies with children. *Am. J. Psychiatry,* 126:884-888.

Conners, C. K., Taylor, E., Meo, G., Kurtz, M. A., and Fournier, M. 1972. Magnesium pemoline and dextroamphetamine: A controlled study in children with minimal brain dysfunction. *Psychopharmacologia,* 26:321-336.

DiMascio, A. 1971. Psychopharmacology in children. *Massachusetts Journal of Mental Health,* Fall, 1970, Vol. 1, No. 1.

DiMascio, A. 1975. An examination of actual medication usage in retardation institutions: A study of 2,000 cases. In J. G. Langan (chm.), *Workshop on Psychotropic Drugs and the Mentally Retarded.* Symposium presented at the meeting of the American Association on Mental Deficiency, Portland.

Ellis, N. R. 1970. Memory processes in retarded and normals. In N. R. Ellis (ed.),

International Review of Research in Mental Retardation, vol. 4, pp. 1-32. New York: Academic Press.

GADOW, K. D. 1975. Pills and preschool: Medication usage with young children in special education. Paper presented at the Illinois Council for Exceptional Children, Chicago.

GADOW, K. D. 1976. Psychotropic and anticonvulsant drug usage in early childhood special education programs I. A preliminary report: Prevalence, attitude, and training. Paper presented at the annual meeting of the Council for Exceptional Children, Chicago.

GALLAGHER, C. E. 1970. Federal involvement in the use of behavior modification drugs on grammar school children of the right to privacy inquiry. *Hearing before a Subcommittee of the Committee on Government Operations. House of Representatives, 91st Congress, 2nd Session.* Washington, D.C.: U.S. Government Printing Office, Publication 52-268.

Gary W. v. State of Louisiana. 1976. No. 74 2412 (E. D. Louisiana).

GOODMAN, L. S., and GILMAN, A. 1970. *The Pharmacological Basis of Therapeutics*, 4th Ed. New York: Macmillan.

KRAGER, J. M., and SAFER, D. J. 1974. Type and prevalence of medication used in the treatment of hyperactive children. *N. Eng. J. Med.*, 291:1118-1120.

KUPIETZ, S., BIALER, I., and WINSBERG, B. G. 1972. A behavior rating scale for assessing improvement in behaviorally deviant children: A preliminary investigation. *Am. J. Psychiatry*, 128:1432-1436.

LIPMAN, R. S. 1970. The use of psychopharmacological agents in residential facilities for the retarded. In F. J. Menolascino (ed.), *Psychiatric Approaches to Mental Retardation*, pp. 387-398. New York: Basic Books.

MAYNARD, R. 1970. Omaha pupils given "behavior" drugs. *Washington Post*, June 29.

MOSHER, L. 1975. Pawns in a pill game. *The National Observer*, January 11.

New York State Association for Retarded Children, Inc. v. Nelson Rockefeller, 1975. No. 72 356, 72 357 (E. D. New York).

ROSS, D. M., and ROSS, S. A. 1976. *Hyperactivity: Research, Theory, and Action*. New York: Wiley.

RUSSELL, R. W. 1960. Drugs as tools in behavioral research. In L. Uhr and J. G. Miller (eds.), *Drugs and Behavior*, pp. 19-40. New York: Wiley.

SAFER, D. J., and ALLEN, R. P. 1976. *Hyperactive Children: Diagnosis and Management*. Baltimore: University Park Press.

SCHRAG, P., and DIVOKY, D. 1975. *The Myth of the Hyperactive Child*. New York: Pantheon.

SCOTT, K. G. 1971. Recognition memory: A research strategy and a summary of initial findings. In N. R. Ellis (ed.), *International Review of Research in Mental Retardation*, vol. 5, pp. 84-111. New York: Academic Press.

SCOVILLE, B. 1974. Governmental perspectives in the evaluation and regulation of stimulant drugs for hyperkinetic children. In J. J. Bosco (chm.), *Stimulant Drugs and the Schools: Dimensions of Social Toxicity*. Symposium presented at the Council on Exceptional Children, New York.

SILVERMAN, M., and LEE, P. R. 1974. *Pills, Profits, and Politics*. Berkeley: University of California Press.

SPRAGUE, R. L. 1976a. Counting jars of raspberry jam. In R. P. Anderson and C. G. Halcomb (eds.), *Learning Disability/Minimal Brain Dysfunction Syndrome*, pp. 94-125. Springfield, Ill.: Charles C Thomas.

SPRAGUE, R. L. 1976b. Overview of psychopharmacology for the retarded in the United States. In R. L. Sprague (chm.), *The Use of Pharmacological Agents in Mental Retardation*. Symposium presented at the Fourth International Congress of the

International Association for the Scientific Study of Mental Deficiency, Washington, D.C.

Sprague, R. L., Barnes, K., and Werry, J. S. 1970. Methylphenidate and thioridazine: Learning, reaction time, activity, and classroom behavior in emotionally disturbed children. *Am. J. Orthopsychiatry*, 40:615-628.

Sprague, R. L., Christensen, D. E., and Werry, J. S. 1974. Experimental psychology and stimulant drugs. In C. K. Conners (ed.), *Clinical Use of Stimulant Drugs in Children*, pp. 141-164. The Hague: Excerpta Medica.

Sprague, R. L., and Gadow, K. 1976. Training teachers about psychotropic drugs. *School Review*, 85:109-140.

Sprague, R. L., and Sleator, E. K. 1973. Effects of psychopharmacologic agents on learning disorders. *Pediatr. Clin. North Am.*, 20:719-735.

Sprague, R. L., and Sleator, E. K. 1975. What is the proper dose of stimulant drugs in children? *International Journal of Mental Health*, 4:75-104.

Sprague, R. L., and Sleator, E. K. 1976. Drugs and dosages: Implications for learning disabilities. In R. M. Knights and D. J. Bakker (eds.), *Neuropsychology of Learning Disorders: Theoretical Approaches*. Baltimore: University Park Press.

Sprague, R. L., and Werry, J. S. 1971. Methodology of psychopharmacological studies with the retarded. In N. R. Ellis (ed.), *International Review of Research in Mental Retardation*, vol. 5, pp. 147-219. New York: Academic Press.

Sprague, R. L., and Werry, J. S. 1974. Psychotropic drugs and handicapped children. In L. Mann and D. A. Sabatino (eds.), *The Second Review of Special Education*, pp. 1-50. Philadelphia: JSE Press.

The Wyat case: Implementation of a judicial decree ordering institutional change. 1975. *84 Yale Law Journal*, 1338.

Velie, L. 1976. Is anybody watching? *Reader's Digest*, March, pp. 114-118.

Werry, J. S., and Quay, H. C. 1969. Observing the classroom behavior of elementary school children. *Except. Child.*, 35:461-472.

Werry, J. S., Sprague, R. L., and Cohen, M. N. 1975. Conners' Teacher Rating Scale for use in drug studies with children—An empirical study. *J. Abnorm. Child Psychol.*, 3:217-229.

Winchell, C. A. 1975. The hyperkinetic child: A bibliography of medical, educational, and behavioral studies. Westport, Conn.: Greenwood Press.

Wyatt v. Anderholt. 1974. 503 F. 2d 1305 (5th Cir.).

Zeaman, D., and House, B. J. 1963. The role of attention in retardate discrimination learning. In N. R. Ellis (ed.), *Handbook of Mental Deficiency*, pp. 159-223. New York: McGraw-Hill.

Part IV
RESEARCH ON THE FAMILY

9

Chronic Asthma: A New Approach
to Treatment

RONALD LIEBMAN, M.D.
SALVADOR MINUCHIN, M.D.
LESTER BAKER, M.D.
and
BERNICE ROSMAN, Ph.D.

Introduction and Review of Literature

This paper is concerned with children who develop chronic, severe, relapsing asthma in spite of competent pediatric management. Candidates for parentectomy, they improve after separation from the family but may relapse after returning home (Peshkin and Tuft, 1956; Long et al., 1958; Sperling, 1968; Pinkerton, 1969; Pinkerton and Weaver 1970). We contend that this syndrome, which Peshkin and Tuft (1956) have labeled intractable asthma, represents a psychosomatic disorder in which the primary allergic disorder has been complicated profoundly by emotional factors, especially chronic, unresolved conflicts in the family. These conflicts engender chronic stress that precipitates acute attacks and perpetuates the chronicity of the illness. Therefore, the system of the family is the basic unit to-

These studies were supported in part by U.S.P.H.S. Grants RR #240 and MH #21336. This chapter has been adapted from Liebman, R., Minuchin, S., and Baker, L. 1974. *American Journal of Psychiatry*, 131:535-540.

ward which therapeutic interventions should be directed (Sperling, 1968; Pinkerton, 1969; Grolnick, 1972).

We have identified patterns of family organization and functioning associated with psychosomatic illness in children, and we have developed a therapeutic approach designed to change these patterns (Minuchin et al., 1975). Our results suggest that structural family therapy represents a significant breakthrough in the treatment of this perplexing and frustrating illness.

A review of the literature indicates that children with intractable asthma constitute 10 to 12 percent of children with asthma (Rackemann and Edwards, 1952). Many investigators have reported the importance of intrapsychic, interpersonal, and family factors in the precipitation of the acute attacks and in the development of chronic forms of the disorder (Knapp and Nemetz, 1957; Weblin, 1963; McLean and Ching, 1973; French, 1939; French and Alexander, 1941; Coolidge, 1956; Cohen, 1971; Mohr et al., 1963). The success of parentectomy in alleviating the symptoms indicates the effect of the family on the clinical course of intractable asthma. The studies of Long et al. (1958), which found that 18 of 19 hospitalized asthmatic children showed no evidence of respiratory distress after exposure to high concentrations of their own house dust, and of Owen (1963), which showed that hospitalized asthmatic children responded to tape recordings of their mothers' voices with more changes in their patterns of respiratory activity than a control group, provide supporting evidence. Pinkerton's work presents excellent arguments for reducing intrafamilial stress to maintain clinical improvement (Pinkerton, 1967, 1969, 1972; Pinkerton and Weaver, 1970). This paper will describe a family-oriented treatment program which has proven successful in the treatment of chronic, severe asthma.

CHRONIC SEVERE ASTHMA IN THE FAMILY

We have observed that the parents of patients with chronic, severe asthma tend to be intrinsically overdependent, especially on physicians. Frequently, the parents imagine the doctor to be a powerful person who possesses certain magical qualities that will enable him to cure their child. The family system exerts a powerful pull on the pediatrician, drawing him into a position of overinvolvement in which his attempts to deal with the child's symptoms meet with little success. From the families we have treated, we have delineated the following course of events associated with the development of chronic severe asthma in the family.

A significant factor is the manner in which the family system, especially the parents, responds to the diagnosis of asthma. In addition, the quality of the relationship between the parents and the physician and the intensity with which they respond to his suggestions concerning management influence the course of the illness. The greater the dependency of the parents on the physician, plus the presence of certain family characteristics (to be described below), the greater the possibility for the development of the psychosomatic syndrome of chronic, severe, relapsing asthma.

After the occurrence of significant allergic symptoms and/or an attack of wheezing, the family's pediatrician suggests to the parents that they see an allergist for a more thorough evaluation of their child. After taking a detailed history and obtaining the results of skin tests, cultures, blood studies, and x-rays, the parents are usually told that the primary problem is one of allergic hypersensitivity and hyperreactivity to offending allergens. Commonly, the patient is found to be allergic to house dust, certain foods, certain pollens and molds, and animal fur or dander. The importance of infection as a precipitating and perpetuating factor is stressed, and some comment is usually made indicating that strenuous physical activity may precipitate an attack of asthma. The parents are cautioned that attacks frequently occur in the early-morning hours after the patient has gone to sleep.

Following this introduction, all or part of the following therapeutic regimen may be outlined for the patient and parents: The house must be thoroughly cleaned and kept as dust-free as possible on a daily basis; certain foods must be avoided because of their potential allergenic nature; frequently, household pets have to be given away; a program of desensitization is recommended to decrease the allergy to pollens and molds; the patient's peer-group relations and extracurricular activities are curtailed; and it is recommended that the patient avoid competitive sports, including physical education classes in school (Nelson, 1964).

Obviously, this regimen affects the entire family. The most significant effects are experienced by the parents. When they are told that the child might have asthmatic attacks during the night, the mother may decide to leave the bedroom doors open to insure that someone will hear the slightest wheeze. The open door policy results in a loss of privacy and autonomy for all the family members. The tension and anxiety that arise at bedtime decrease the frequency and gratification of sexual relationships. The mother may become overinvolved with the patient to the extent of neglecting the needs of other family members. Her overinvolvement with the patient usually occurs at the expense of the marital relationship. If the family remains intact, significant conflict and stress develop between the parents, and between the patient and the more peripheral parent. The patient experiences guilt because he feels, in some way, responsible for the problems between his parents. However, parents and siblings have been cautioned not to upset or overstimulate the patient. Thus, the hostility and resentment are submerged, to be acted out in covert, self-defeating, maladaptive patterns.

The entire family becomes organized around emergencies associated with the symptoms of the patient in order to get him to the doctor or hospital as quickly as possible. As a result, the father's work record suffers and his future may be compromised. Family vacations and trips become significant problems because of the possibility of an acute attack. The parents rarely go away by themselves because they are afraid that the patient may become ill.

The siblings of the patient usually feel neglected. They harbor a great deal of resentment toward the patient, which is generally suppressed. The siblings tend to act out their resentment at home or school to get their parents' attention. There is an increase of sibling rivalry. The patient is usually excluded from the activities planned by the siblings.

The effects of the traditional regimen on the patient are significant. He becomes labeled as a special, sick, weak child. This leads to the development of low self-esteem, a decrease in self-confidence, and a decrease in his ability to cope with and solve problems. Significant secondary handicaps in the areas of educational underachievement and emotional and behavioral maladjustment have been reported (Pless and Roghmann, 1971). As a result of parental overprotectiveness, his autonomy and independence are constricted. He may be restricted from age-appropriate activities, which results in partial isolation and alienation from his sibship and peer group. His interpersonal relationships in the home, school, and community are impaired.

The patient's special role in the family depends on the presence of his symptoms, and he has tremendous power to manipulate the family through his symptoms. Frequently, he is not appropriately disciplined because his parents are afraid to upset him. This has maladaptive consequences for the patient, the parents, the relationship between the patient and his siblings, and the relationships between the parents and the siblings. The family system that emerges is characterized by hostility, tension, frustration, and anxiety. These feelings have to be avoided within the context of the family, however, to protect the patient from being overstimulated.

If asthmatic attacks continue, the physician may assume that the patient is not following the details of the treatment program, or that the parents, especially the mother, are not having the child follow the regimen. Consequently, a more vigorous attempt is made to get the family to follow the regimen. If acute attacks still occur, the physician may conclude that emotional factors are causing the child to fail to respond, and a psychiatric evaluation is recommended. At this point, the suppressed frustration, anger, and anxiety of the family are transferred to the child psychiatrist. The traditional, one-to-one, dynamically-oriented approach may fail with the chronic, asthmatic patient (Sperling, 1968; Purcell, Bernstein, and Bukantz, 1961) because it intensifies the role of the patient as the sick member of the family, neglecting the roles of the parents and siblings in perpetuating the symptoms. It supports the patient's role as the symptom bearer for the family. If traditional one-to-one psychotherapy fails, the child psychiatrist refers the family back to the pediatrician. Having tried everything, the pediatrician often concludes that it is contraindicated for the patient to remain with his family. He may suggest that parentectomy is the only remaining method which might reverse the chronic relapsing course of the illness.

The parents' feelings of impotence, frustration, and hopelessness result in their agreeing to parentectomy—the process whereby the sick family member is removed from the family and transplanted to a safe place where the family no longer has to deal with him or their ambivalent feelings toward him. As a result of parentectomy, the family is given the message that it has a noxious, deleterious influence on the patient. This engenders even more guilt and frustration on the part of the family. The patient is angry and resentful toward his family because of separation. Parentectomy amplifies the feelings of hopelessness and helplessness that pervade the entire family, and particularly the patient who is now physically removed from his main source of security and nurturance. The process of removal crystallizes in the patient the formation of a profound, negative self-image because he perceives himself as a defective, inferior, sick, helpless, weak person who is so repulsive to his family that he has to be removed from it. This perception unfortunately is supported by the behavior of the family. The child has become a medical invalid who is crippled by his symptoms.

Thus, we see parentectomy as a process that is emotionally traumatic and deleterious to the family and to the patient in particular. We have developed an alternative to parentectomy, which enables the child with chronic, severe asthma to stay at home with his family where he can grow and develop in an age-appropriate fashion. This alternative—structural family therapy—consists of changing the structure and functioning of the family to eliminate the factors that reinforce the symptoms and perpetuate the chronicity of the illness.

CHARACTERISTICS OF THE PSYCHOSOMATIC FAMILY

On the basis of our clinical studies, we have observed that the development of severe psychosomatic symptoms in a child is related to the presence of certain patterns of family organization and functioning which have the following interactional characteristics (Minuchin et al., 1975):

1. *Enmeshment*: Family members are overinvolved with and overresponsive to one another. Attempted changes by any member stimulate a chain of events to maintain the status quo and prevent change from occurring. Family members intrude upon each other's thoughts, feelings, activities, and communications. There is a decrease in the autonomy and privacy of individual family members, and the generational boundaries between parents and children are weak and easily crossed. Interpersonal boundaries that define where one person leaves off and the other begins are also weak, resulting in a confusion of roles.

2. *Overprotectiveness*: The family members have a high degree of concern for each other, with nurturing and protective responses being constantly elicited and supplied. Parental overprotectiveness results in a decrease in the extrafamilial relationships and activities of the patient. When the patient becomes sick, the entire family becomes organized around his care, often submerging intrafamilial conflicts in the process.

3. *Rigidity*: The family often presents itself as being completely normal without any problems except for the patient's medical problems. Therefore, they deny the need for change within the family system and they preserve accustomed patterns of interaction and behavior.

4. *Lack of conflict resolution*: There is a low threshold for overt conflict in these families. Confrontations involving differences of opinion and issues of autonomy and control are avoided or diffused. Consequently, there is a chronic state of submerged, unresolved conflict with the stress and tension associated with it. The child with severe psychosomatic symptoms plays a vital part in the family's avoidance of conflict. The experience of being able to protect the family, especially the parents, from conflict by way of symptoms is a powerful reinforcement to the patient. In addition, the sibling

subsystem may reinforce the symptoms as part of a protective and/or a scapegoating system.

5. *The patient is involved in parental conflict*: In these families, in which generational boundaries between the parents and the children are weak and easily crossed, the child's symptoms function as a conflict-avoidance, detouring mechanism, especially in connection with the detouring of spouse conflicts. Submerged conflicts that threaten the stability of the spouse dyad, the marriage, and the maintenance of an intact family system remain submerged by total concentration on the symptoms of the patient. The patient is brought, and to a certain extent brings himself, into the spouse dyad to form a triad through which the conflict between the spouses can be detoured. Thus, the patient's symptoms protect the family structure and are reinforced by that structure.

Two of our families illustrate this point. A pattern existed in which the patient would begin to develop symptoms Friday evening or Saturday morning. By Saturday evening, the parents would have to take the patient to the emergency room for treatment, a process which involved several hours. Previously, when the parents had gone out Saturday evening, they had occasionally abused alcohol and returned home to verbally and/or physically abuse each other. The development of acute attacks that required a trip to the hospital protected the parents. Thus, the parents did not go out socially and were preoccupied with the medical status of the patient. As long as the spouse conflicts remained unresolved, the symptoms of the patient would persist.

A typical consequence of the conflict-detouring process is the dysfunctional set. A dysfunctional set is a pattern of defective or ineffective communication between two or more people that results in a lack of resolution of disagreements and the perpetuation of the stress and tension that exist between them. Frequently, the dysfunctional set is a part of the family system in which there is a strong alliance between mother and patient with an excluded, angry, peripheral father. In this system, the dysfunctional set consists of the

TABLE 1

Summary of 14 Cases of Intractable Asthma

Patient	Sex-Age	Age at Onset	Steroid Dependent	*Clinical Severity	Duration Family Therapy	*Current Status	Duration of follow-up (post-therapy)
1	F-8	3 yrs.	yes	Grade 3	7 months	Grade 1	3 yrs. 10 mos.
2	F-12	3 yrs.	yes	Grade 3	6 months	Grade 1	4 yrs.
3	F-11	15 mos.	yes	Grade 3	9 months	Grade 1	2 yrs. 7 mos.
4	M-13	11 yrs.	no	Grade 3	5 months	Grade 1	5 yrs.
5	M-15	18 mos.	yes	Grade 4	22 months	Grade 2	4 yrs.
6	M-8	6 yrs.	yes	Grade 3	8 months	Grade 1	3 yrs. 6 mos.
7	M-11	3½ yrs.	yes	Grade 3	6 months	Grade 1	2 yrs.
8	F-11	1 yr.	yes	Grade 3	11 months	Grade 1	3 yrs. 9 mos.
9	M-12	18 mos.	yes	Grade 4	8 months	Grade 2	2 yrs. 8 mos.
10	F-6	6 yrs.	no	Grade 2	6 months	Grade 1	2 yrs. 7 mos.
11	M-7	2 yrs.	yes	Grade 3	12 months	Grade 1	2 yrs. 3 mos.
12	M-10	7 yrs.	yes	Grade 4	20 months	Grade 2	18 months
13	M-15	5 yrs.	yes	Grade 4	11 months	Grade 2	1 year
14	M-10	3½ yrs.	yes	Grade 3	14 months	Grade 1	2 yrs. 7 mos.

* Pinkerton and Weaver (1970) Scale for Evaluation of Clinical Severity of Asthma

Grade 1: No school loss, mild attacks, occasional need for bronchodilator.
Grade 2: Days off school, mild to moderate attacks, need for regular bronchodilator.
Grade 3: Weeks off school, more prolonged and severe attacks, need for steroid in addition to bronchodilator.
Grade 4: More than 50 percent school loss, persistent symptoms, need for special schooling, need for regular steroid therapy.

father and the patient. The presence of a specific dysfunctional set is supported by other dysfunctional relationships in the family, particularly between the parents. It is manifested by the patient's becoming upset and developing an asthmatic attack when the father disciplines or criticizes him. The wheezing drives the father away and calls the mother and siblings in to protect the child. Then, the family organizes itself around the task of taking the patient to the hospital.

The characteristics of the psychosomatogenic family are important because they constitute the foundation and direction for family therapy aimed at correcting dysfunctional family patterns and disengaging the children from the arena of spouse conflict.

REVIEW OF PATIENTS

We have evaluated, treated, and followed 14 families with a chronic asthmatic child (Table 1). Since the time of diagnosis, they have failed to respond to competent, adequate medical management during a period of several months to several years. All have had significant, severe asthmatic symptoms and have been maintained on chronic steroids, bronchodilators, and Intermittent Positive-Presence Breathing (IPPB) treatments. They have had vigorous courses of allergic desensitization and therapeutic trials of several different bronchodilators. Eight of the patients had individually oriented psychotherapy or counseling prior to referral. The patients had lost significant amounts of time from school and had had several acute attacks requiring emergency treatment and/or hospitalization. Several aspects of their physical and personality development had suffered because of their isolation from school and peer group, and the effects of chronic illness and steroid administration. Before referral, several of the parents had been presented with the possibility of parentectomy in an attempt to alleviate the severe, crippling, asthmatic symptoms. In all cases, the referring allergist felt that emotional problems in the patient and/or within the family were a major factor contributing to the severity and chronicity of the asthma.

The Treatment Program

General Principles

Treatment of the child within the context of his family frequently engenders a significant amount of anxiety in the family members, which can be used to motivate the family to enter therapy, in spite of the occasional occurrence of an initial period of resistance to therapy. There is a need to shift responsibility for the care of the patient away from the pediatrician and the hospital, and back to the family. Ultimately, the patient will be able to assume more age-appropriate responsibility for the care of his illness.

Initially, the transfer of responsibility is met with resistance by the parents who try to increase their dependency on the pediatrician. These initial problems must be overcome if the family psychiatrist is to gain entrance to the family system where he will transiently function as a catalyst to effect changes.

In treating these families, we have been able to delineate a consistent importance factor—the willingness and ability of the pediatrician to transfer and share medical authority and responsibility with the family psychiatrist. The pediatrician must support the family psychiatrist and deemphasize some of the aspects of previous medical management. Consequently, this will enable the family psychiatrist to gradually return more responsibility to the parents. As the parents' dependence on the pediatrician decreases, the patient and the parents become increasingly able to cope with the asthmatic symptoms, which results in a significant reduction in emergency visits to the pediatrician or hospital.

Since the symptoms of the patient occur within the context of the family and are reinforced by the family, it is logical and appropriate to consider the family the basic unit that requires change. Specifically, the structure and functioning of the family system must be changed to enable the patient to change his role as the symptom bearer of the family. Once this is achieved, the patient will have more freedom to establish meaningful peer-group relationships and extrafamilial activities.

The general characteristics of structural family therapy (Minuchin, 1974) are as follows:

1. The term, structural, refers to the concept of the family as a system consisting of various subsystems. In the treatment of psychosomatic illness in children, the parental and child subsystems and the generational boundaries that separate them are most important.

2. It is systemic because it is assumed that the patient will not be able to give up his symptoms or change his role in the family unless the structure and functioning of the family system are changed.

3. It is goal-directed because therapeutic interventions are directed at correcting dysfunctional behavior patterns in the family.

4. Therapeutically, it is concerned with the present and immediate future, not the past.

5. It is based on observable, transactional, interpersonal processes between and among family members; it is not based on psychoanalytic concepts of the development of psychopathology.

The success of the structural family therapy approach is manifested by the clinical improvement of the asthmatic child as a result of therapeutic interventions aimed at changing the structure and functioning of the family. We consider a successful outcome to be constituted by the following: elimination or significant alleviation of severe symptoms resulting in significant reduction of emergency trips to the pediatrician or hospital; elimination of chronic dependency on steroids, IPPB treatments, or nebulizers; restoration of normal physical activity and age-appropriate peer-group relations; a normal school or work attendance record; and the *alteration of dysfunctional family patterns that reinforced and perpetuated the patient's symptoms.*

Goals of Treatment

The weekly outpatient family therapy sessions are organized into three phases depending on the goals to be accomplished in each phase. Phase 1 is concerned with the alleviation of the symptoms of asthma to prevent the use of the patient as a means of detouring family conflicts. Once the symptoms are reduced, there is more freedom and flexibility available to promote change within the family. Phase 2 consists of identifying and changing those patterns in the family and extrafamilial environment that tended to exacerbate and perpetuate the severe symptoms. Phase 3 consists of interventions to change the structure and functioning of the family system to promote lasting disengagement of the patient in order to prevent a recurrence of the symptoms or the development of a new symptom bearer.

The pediatrician assumes a significant role in the early phase of family therapy. It is important for the family psychiatrist and the pediatrician to discuss the treatment program and to develop a cooperative working relationship of mutual support, respect, and confidence. The pediatrician should be present during the first family therapy session to state explicitly that medical management has not been successful in the past and that, in the future, medical management will be deemphasized. This will show the family that he supports and agrees with the family psychiatrist's desire to transfer more of the responsibility for the management of symptoms to the patient and the parents.

The specific goals in the early phases are as follows: to desensitize the patient and the family to the problems of asthma, instilling the possibility for hope and symptom improvement; to help the parents and the patient to avoid emergency treatments and/or hospitalizations by increasing their ability to cope with precipitating stressful situations; to change the role and status of the patient in the family into being an equal, healthy, functioning member who receives no special treatment or privileges; and to enable the family to accept the patient as a more healthy, autonomous member.

Treatment Process and Techniques

The first step is to stop the patient from functioning as a detourer of family conflicts by helping him to decrease the intensity and frequency of acute attacks. This is accomplished by using different strategies and interventions. The work of Luparello emphasizes the importance of the patient's expectations, suggestibility, and conditioning regarding the precipitation and treatment of acute attacks (Luparello et al., 1968; Luparello et al., 1970; Luparello et al., 1971). LaScola reported on treatment of acute attacks by teaching the patient muscle relaxation exercises (LaScola, 1968). The reports on the principles and use of behavior modification and biofeedback training raise the possibility for increased voluntary control of asthmatic symptoms (Miller, 1969; Gaarder, 1971; Alexander, 1972; Alexander, Miklick, and Hershkoff, 1972; Heim, Blaser, and Waidelich, 1972). We have been able to use these principles by teaching the patient a series of deep-breathing exercises at the first sign of bronchoconstriction, which is usually a "squeak" at the end of expiration. The exercises are done until the squeak disappears and the dyspnea is relieved. Although behavior modification and breathing exercises are effective in decreasing the patient's symptoms, they do nothing to change the context of the patient's family in which the symptoms originated and are reinforced. Therefore, behavior modification and biofeedback exercises *alone* will not prevent relapses after active therapy is stopped.

We use the process of teaching the exercises to the patient as a technique for changing the structural relationships within the family system. For instance, in a family in which the patient is closely allied with the mother and the father is peripheral, with a dysfunctional set existing between father and patient, we assign the father the daily task of practicing the breathing exercises with the patient. The mother is advised to help her husband learn to relate more effectively to the patient, but not to exclude or undermine him by taking this responsibility away from him. This decreases the coalition between mother and patient; it modifies the dysfunctional set between father and patient and between the parents; it changes the role of the father in the family by increasing his involvement in a constructive manner; and it shifts the relationship between the parents to a more mutually supportive, goal-directed level.

The increased control of symptoms gives the patient and parents hope and optimism. The changes in family relationships increase the emotional distance between the patient and his parents, facilitating disengagement of the patient from spouse conflicts. It also expedites the return of the patient to the child subsystem of the family, which prepares the patient for increased peer-group activities in the future.

To provide the patient with an increased feeling of mastery and increased autonomy, one can establish an operant-reinforcement paradigm in which increased accessibility to age-appropriate, peer-group activities is made contingent on progressive symptom reduction. This is an effective therapeutic strategy because symptom reduction will provide increased freedom and autonomy for the entire family.

The parents should be instructed on emergency treatment for an asthmatic attack at home and provided with adrenalin and syringes. If an acute attack fails to respond to muscle relaxation, the more peripheral parent is given the task of calling the pediatrician to get instructions on administering the appropriate amount of adrenalin. This prevents an emergency trip to the pediatrician's office or the hospital. It is an effective strategy because it increases the competence of the parents in dealing with their sick child and strengthens generational boundaries in the family. The parents are told that if they work together in a mutually supportive way, they will succeed in helping the patient master the symptoms. This uncovers pathogenic coalitions, power struggles, and dysfunctional sets, and provides an opportunity to deal with them in the family therapy sessions.

Other general guidelines are as follows:

1. To search for dysfunctional sets that produce stress and precipitate acute attacks and convert them into functional sets.

2. To change pathogenic relationships that are maintained by the patient's symptoms.

3. To uncover concrete problems (school, peer group, etc.) that involve the patient's siblings. Frequently, these problems have not been attended to by the parents because of their preoccupation with the patient. One must focus on one problem at a time, with one sibling, and instruct the parents to organize a plan to help the sibling solve the particular problem. They must follow through with every

detail of their plan, and they are advised to have private discussions each evening in their bedroom. This modifies the dysfunctional set between the parents. Although this problem-solving approach may appear superficial, it is effective in removing the patient as the sole symptom bearer in the family, decreasing his centrality and power to manipulate the family. Furthermore, it renders the patient less deviant and less isolated from his siblings because all of the children now have problems that demand equal attention from the parents. It forces the parents to work together in a mutually supportive way, preventing the patient's symptoms from splitting the spouse dyad. The parents' experience of helping their children cope with their problems increases the parents' self-esteem and self-confidence as the executive heads of the family.

4. To return the patient to the child subsystem and strengthen the boundaries between the parental and child subsystems. One must confront the parents about special treatment of the patient, which has allowed him to avoid household responsibilities and appropriate discipline. The patient must not be treated differently from his siblings and must be seen as an equal, responsible member of the child subsystem.

5. To disengage the parents from an enmeshed, overprotective relationship with the patient. One begins by having the parents plan to go out one evening a week, leaving the children home with a baby-sitter. The next step is to have the parents plan to go away overnight or for a weekend. It is most important to clarify and organize a plan of action to decrease parental anxiety if an emergency develops when the parents are not home. If the parents have an open-door policy in the bedroom, they are encouraged to secure privacy by keeping the doors closed. Simultaneously, one enlists the parents' support to encourage the patient to develop age-appropriate, peer-group, and sibling relationships and activities. The parents are given the task of arranging with school authorities for the patient's resumption of physical education classes and encouraging his participation in extra-curricular activities.

There is a constant redefinition of the problems away from the scapegoating, conflict-detouring process that centralized and reinforced the patient's asthmatic symptoms. Instead, the family becomes involved in and concerned about interpersonal transactional issues within the family system. Finally, the emphasis shifts to activities outside of the family, involving the school and peer group. One must employ a broad-based, flexible approach to promote constructive changes in the system constituted by the patient, his family, and the extrafamilial environment.

As the patient's symptoms decrease, there is a gradual increase in the stress between the parents associated with the surfacing of long-submerged marital conflicts. At this point, the therapist must shift his emphasis to the spouse dyad to resolve chronic conflicts that have been detoured by concern with the patient's symptoms. By working to resolve or alleviate the problems of the spouse dyad, one sows the seeds for preventing a recurrence of symptoms in the patient.

RESULTS

The results of our treatment program can be summarized as follows (Table 1):

1. Family therapy has been successful in alleviating the intensity and frequency of acute attacks of asthma. Although some of the patients have occasional attacks of wheezing, the patients and their families have increased ability to cope with the symptoms, resulting in fewer hospitalizations and fewer emergency visits to the pediatrician.

2. The patients are no longer medical cripples and are less dependent on the daily use of steroids, IPPB treatments, or desensitization programs. Periodically, however, medications are used to treat acute seasonal attacks of wheezing associated with specific allergies.

3. The patients have more normal age-appropriate life-styles associated with markedly improved school attendance, increased peer-group involvement, and increased physical activities.

4. There have been associated positive changes in the functioning and interpersonal relationships of the siblings and parents.

Based on our experience and the results of this program, we consider a family-oriented approach to be effective in the treatment of chronic, severe asthma in children.

REFERENCES

ALEXANDER, A. B. 1972. Systematic relaxation and flow rates in asthmatic children: Relationship to emotional precipitants and anxiety. *J. Psychosom. Res.*, 16:405-410.

ALEXANDER, A. B., MIKLICK, D. R., and HERSHKOFF, H. 1972. The immediate effects of systematic relaxation training on peak expiratory flow rates in asthmatic children. *Psychosom. Med.*, 34:388-394.

BIOFEEDBACK IN ACTION. *Medical World News*, March 9, 1973. pp. 47-60.

COHEN, S. I. 1971. Psychological factors in asthma: A review of their etiological and therapeutic significance. *Postgrad. Med. J.*, 47:533-540.

COOLIDGE, J. C. 1956. Asthma in mother and child as a special type of intercommunication. *Am. J. Orthopsychiatry*, 26:165-178.

FRENCH, T. M. 1939. Psychogenic factors in asthma. *Am. J. Psychiatry*, 96:87-101.

FRENCH, T. M., and ALEXANDER, R. 1941. Psychogenic factors in bronchial asthma. *Psychosom. Med. Monograph IV*. Washington, D.C.: National Research Council.

GAARDER, K. 1971. Control of states of consciousness, I and II. *Arch. Gen. Psychiatry*, 25:429-444.

GROLNICK, L. 1972. A family perspective of psychosomatic factors in illness: A review of the literature. *Family Process*, 11:457-486.

HEIM, E., BLASER, A., and WAIDELICH, E. 1972. Dyspnea: Psychophysiologic relationship. *Psychosom. Med.*, 34:405-423.

KNAPP, P. H., and NEMETZ, S. J. 1957. Personality variation in bronchial asthma: A study of 40 patients. *Psychosom. Med.*, 19:443-465.

LASCOLA, R. L. 1968. Hypnosis with children. In D. B. Cheek and L. M. Lecron (eds.), *Clinical Hypnotherapy*, pp. 201-211. New York: Grune & Stratton.

LONG, R. T., LAMONT, J. H., WHIPPLE, B., BANDLER, L., BLOOM, G., BURGIN, L., and JESSNER, L. 1958. A psychosomatic study of allergic and emotional factors in children with asthma. *Am. J. Psychiatry*, 114:890-899.

LUPARELLO, T. J., LYONS, H. A., BLEECKER, E. R., and McFADDEN, E. 1968. Influences of suggestion on airway reactivity in asthmatic subjects. *Psychosom. Med.*, 30: 819-825.

LUPARELLO, T. J., LEIST, N., LOURIE, C. H., and SWEET, P. 1970. The interaction of psychologic stimuli and pharmacologic agents on airway reactivity in asthmatic subjects. *Psychosom. Med.*, 32:509-513.

LUPARELLO, T. J., McFADDEN, E. R., LYONS, H. A., and BLEECKER, E. R. 1971. Psychologic factors and bronchial asthma. *N.Y. State J. Med.*, 71:2161-2165.

McLEAN, J. A., and CHING, A. Y. T. 1973. Follow-up study of relationships between family situation and bronchial asthma in children. *J. Am. Acad. Child Psychiatry*, 12:142-161.

MILLER, N. E. 1969. Learning of visceral and glandular responses. *Science*, 163:434-445.

MINUCHIN, S. 1974. *Families and Family Therapy: A Structural Approach*. Boston: Harvard University Press.

MINUCHIN, S., BAKER, L., ROSMAN, B., LIEBMAN, R., MILMAN, L., and TODD, T. 1975. A conceptual model of psychosomatic illness in children. *Arch. Gen. Psychiatry,* 32:1031-1038.

MOHR, C. J., TAUSEND, H., and SELESNICK, S. 1963. Studies of eczema and asthma in the preschool child. *J. Am. Acad. Child Psychiatry,* 2:271-291.

NELSON, W. E. 1964. *Textbook of Pediatrics.* Philadelphia: Saunders.

OWEN, F. W. 1963. Patterns of respiratory disturbance in asthmatic children evoked by the stimulus of the mother's voice. *Acta Psychotherapy,* 11:228-241.

PESHKIN, M. M., and TUFT, H. S. 1956. Rehabilitation of the intractable asthmatic child by the institutional approach. *Quarterly Review of Pediatrics,* 11:7-9.

PINKERTON, P. 1967. Correlating physiologic with psychodynamic data in the study and management of childhood asthma. *J. Psychosom. Res.,* 11:95-99.

PINKERTON, P. 1969. Pathophysiology and psychopathology as codeterminants of pharmaco-therapeutic response in childhood asthma. In A. Pletscher and A. Marino (eds.), *Psychotropic Drugs in Internal Medicine,* pp. 115-127. Amsterdam: Excerpta Medica Foundation.

PINKERTON, P., and WEAVER, C. M. 1970. Childhood asthma. In O. Hill (ed.), *Psychosomatic Medicine,* pp. 81-104. London: Butterworths.

PINKERTON, P. 1972. The psychosomatic approach in pediatrics. *Br. Med. J.,* 3:462-464.

PLESS, I. B., and ROGHMANN, K. J. 1971. Chronic illness and its consequences: Observations based on 3 epidemiologic surveys. *J. Pediatr.,* 79:351-359.

PURCELL, K., BERNSTEIN, L., and BUKANTZ, S. C. 1961. A comparison of rapidly remitting and steroid-dependent asthmatic children. *Psychosomatic Medicine,* 23:305-310.

RACKEMANN, F. M., and EDWARDS, M. D. 1952. Asthma in children (a follow-up study). *N. Eng. J. Med.,* 246:815-823.

SPERLING, M. 1968. Asthma in children: An evaluation of concept and therapies. *J. Am. Acad. Child Psychiatry,* 7:44-58.

WEBLIN, J. E. 1963. Pathogenesis in asthma: An appraisal with a view to family research. *Br. J. Med. Psychol.,* 36:211-225.

10

Children at Risk for Psychosis and Their Families: Approaches to Prevention

HENRY GRUNEBAUM, M.D.

Children who live in homes with a psychotic parent have been, and continue to be, of growing interest to researchers and great concern to clinicians because they are likely to develop psychological, social, and educational difficulties. These children offer the opportunity to study precursor variables and environmental conditions that predispose to future psychopathology before the compounding effects of illness and its treatment (Garmezy, 1974a). The focus of most of the research has been on etiology, and there has been comparatively little interest in applying our present knowledge about such children to design effective prevention. It therefore seems an important task to make clinically relevant studies that otherwise would be of no value to the subjects who collaborated in the investigations; it is well known that research reports tend to gather dust in files instead of being used to influence clinical practice.

I should like to acknowledge the contributions of my associates and the meaningfulness of our association in this work which is a truly shared endeavor: Justin Weiss, Bertram Cohler, David Gallant, Carol Hartman, Enid Gamer, Carol Kauffman, and Donna Robbins.

In addition, I should like to acknowledge the contribution of Lyman Wynne whose support, friendship, and thoughtful comments have been of inestimable value, and my debt to Norman Garmezy whose comprehensive reviews have made my task much easier.

This paper is eclectic and suggestive rather than comprehensive or definitive. It attempts to use our present knowledge of children at risk for psychosis to develop avenues for preventive clinical interventions. For these purposes, it seems most useful to define the population at risk rather broadly. Thus, I will discuss two groups of children who are at risk for future mental illness: (1) those who may be detectible because of their behavior; and (2) those children who are at risk genetically and environmentally because they have a psychotic parent. In addition, I will discuss the influence of the attitudes of mental health professionals on vulnerable children and conclude with some practical suggestions for changes in current practice.

Clearly, if one is to intervene preventively with children who are at risk, it is necessary to be able to identify such children—to find an identifiable precursor attribute. Garmezy (1975) has suggested certain criteria that may be used to identify such a characteristic or variable. He notes that: (1) the variable should be present at all stages of the development of the psychopathology and most in evidence when the disorder is manifest; (2) that it should be found in any given population in proportion to the anticipated incidence of the disorder in the population; (3) that it should be relatively stable in any given child, neither evanescent nor dependent entirely on the child's level of motivation; and finally, (4) that it should be a fundamental disposition that relates to competent functioning. Our research (Grunebaum et al., 1974; Gamer and Grunebaum, 1976; Gamer et al., unpublished; Cohler et al., in press), as well as that of other workers, suggests that an attentional parameter is a possible precursor attribute in individuals at risk. It has also been suggested by Wynne and Singer (1963) and Wynne (1967, 1968, in press) that faulty family communication patterns may define families whose members are at risk.

At present, however, no definitive marker variable has been identified. In addition, because the focus of the research on high-risk children has been on the development of schizophrenia in certain children, less attention has been paid to the outcome for the other children in the population at risk whose deficits may be less dramatic but whose lives are nonetheless impaired. Bleuler (1974) has noted that growing up in a family with a psychotic parent may blight one's life even if the outcome is not psychosis. He quotes one man who had a psychotic mother: "When you have gone through that . . . you can never really be happy."

Perhaps the simplest way to learn about the characteristics of children at high risk for developing psychosis is to study the childhood of adults who are psychotic. This approach suffers from the limitation that the data one would like to have usually have not been recorded. However, an excellent example of such a "follow-back" study was conducted by Watt (1972, in press) and Watt et al. (1970), who used very comprehensive school records in a suburban town near Boston to determine the childhood characteristics of 54 children who later became schizophrenic. The differences between the behavior of these children and their 143 matched controls were marked and distinct in the two sexes. The boys were negativistic, egocentric, unpleasant, antisocial, and cheerless, while the girls were primarily quiet, immature, and introverted, though also egocentric; and about 25 percent of the girls were extremely passive. There were frequent references to the emotional immaturity of the children: "crying with the slightest provocation, insensitivity to the feelings of others, temper tantrums, and delayed development" (Watt, 1976). This finding that preschizophrenic males tend to be antisocial while females tend to be socially aloof is supported by other work as reviewed by Rolf and Harig (1974). Watt also found that there was a small number of exceptionally bright and industrious girls who later became schizophrenic. His study showed that the high-risk boys and the high-risk girls experienced a higher incidence of parental deaths and physical handicaps than their controls. While Watt found identifiable characteristics of preschizophrenic children, unfortunately these are also present in a considerable number of the controls. Using all of his criteria and weighing them appropriately, Watt found one could predict 34 of the 54 schizophrenics and 105 of the 143 controls, but one would also diagnose 38 controls as schizophrenic, and miss 20 schizophrenics.

Here, nevertheless, recognition of these characteristics is the beginning of clinical intervention. Clearly, it is possible to help teachers to be aware of difficult and disagreeable boys and of unstable and introverted girls and to offer these children help. Perhaps some of the children who manifested the above characteristics in high school had received help, either formal or informal, psychiatric or lay, planned or unplanned, which prevented their entering the group of psychotics who were studied. Eventually we may learn enough about precursor attributes either of the child or of his family so that intervention efforts can be efficient and effective.

Another group of children who are probably at high risk for developing psychosis as adults are those who seek or are brought for psychiatric help in adolescence. Here the proportion who will eventually become psychotic is unknown, but the characteristics of these children and their families seem similar to those of many young adult schizophrenics and their families. Adolescents with asocial, withdrawn behavior seem to be particularly at risk and are more disturbed on follow-up. They and their families resemble most closely the enmeshed families of schizophrenics. Rodnick and Goldstein (Goldstein et al., 1968; Rodnick and Goldstein, 1972; Goldstein, 1975) have conducted a series of studies on this group while offering them psychotherapeutic intervention, which has been particularly focused on the families' transactional style.

In their studies, certain families of disturbed adolescents seemed to require far more therapeutic assistance than others and "absorbed" it with less change. They were characterized by little responsiveness of the members to each other, centrality of the disturbed offspring in the sessions, and cover-up of intraparental conflicts. It should be noted that while Goldstein and Rodnick (op. cit.) worked solely with intact families, they found the most disturbed families quite resistant to change, as manifested both by their noncooperativeness and their ability to generate crises that took precedence over learning. Nonetheless, some improvement was possible in many instances. This work suggests that therapeutic efforts with disturbed adolescents, particularly if the therapy is family-focused, are likely to be useful, although difficult.

Thus far, I have discussed children who are at risk for developing psychosis by virtue of behaviors they manifest. As yet, we do not know to what extent these behaviors are learned or are inherited. Now, let us turn to children who are at risk because they come from a family with a psychotic parent. Clearly, these children are at risk both genetically and environmentally. At the outset, it is important to remember that only about 10 percent of the children of a schizophrenic parent become schizophrenic, and that only four percent of schizophrenics report having had a parent with schizophrenia. The group of children who are at risk because they have a psychotic parent is a small subset of the total population of children at risk; what we learn from them may or may not apply to the remaining 96 percent, particularly because genetic rather than environmental factors may be of greatest impact in this group. In addition, Watts' work (in press) suggests that very few poor premorbid schizophrenics come from intact families, yet these are precisely the high risk families which have most often been studied.

Work carried out in Minneapolis by Rolf and Garmezy (Rolf, 1972; Rolf and Garmezy, in press; Garmezy, 1974b) and Rolf and Harig (1974) also supports the view that high risk children are likely to come from broken families. These authors, interestingly, find that classroom peers are better able than teachers to detect which children are sons of schizophrenic women, while the reverse is true for daughters of schizophrenic women.

When confronted with the psychosis of a parent, families cope in different ways. Anthony (1968, 1969, 1970) has reported that some families meet the stress of parental disorder by restitution, growth, and differentiation; other families demonstrate a contagion of breakdown within the family, and an early symbiosis can result in the child's sharing the parent's paralogical ideas. Even in these families, some rallying can be observed. Anthony reports that some families, however, are marked by rout and disintegration, in which children seem severely and adversely affected. On the other hand, Romano (cited in Garmezy, 1974b, p. 84) has reported that in the Rochester study most of the psychotic parents recovered from their illness and were asymptomatic when seen; he concludes from his interviews that appropriate parenting attitudes seem to have been sustained. Thus, Anthony's (op. cit.) inner-city, racially mixed, and often nonintact families of St. Louis with a schizophrenic parent differ from the intact, white, and middle-class families studied in Rochester by Romano.

Our own work suggests that reactive schizophrenic and borderline schizophrenic women have maternal attitudes similar to mothers in the control group, while process schizophrenic women manifest far more denial of parental concerns and differ in other ways from normals (Cohler et al., 1968; Cohler, Weiss, and Grunebaum, 1970). In addition, the work of Rodnick and Goldstein (1972) suggests that the schizophrenic mothers differ among themselves. Their studies indicate that women who are older and have older children tend to be on the good premorbid end of the schizophrenic continuum, and that these mothers return to the status of being better caregivers more rapidly after an illness than do the poor premorbid mothers who are younger and have younger children at the onset of the illness.

Let us return to preventive intervention in families in which there is a psychotic mother. Here I shall describe the studies of my colleagues and myself (Grunebaum, 1975; Grunebaum et al., 1975b), for as yet no other investigators have reported the results of their therapeutic efforts. Our work in this area began in 1960 when a 14-month-old boy, "Teddy," joined his psychotic mother on the wards of the Massachusetts Mental Health Center. Subsequently we facilitated many other such "joint admissions" and learned the importance of the voluntary and thoughtful participation of each of the participants in this venture: the mother, the father, the ward staff, and the physician. A series of studies of joint admission demonstrated the striking lack of attention that had hitherto been given to the children of psychotic mothers; often the chart did not even mention their names and ages while describing the mother's childhood and her sibship at length. We found that usually those responsible for her psychiatric care had played no role in what happened to her children during her admission and found that often, during her hospitalization, her children experienced multiple moves and separations.

It was not possible, for obvious reasons, to carry out a study of the effect on the children of joint admission with random assignment to groups. One cannot suggest that a family participate in a joint admission and then not allow them to do so. However, a study that compared children who joined their mothers in the hospital to carefully matched mothers and children who did not, demonstrated that the joint-admission children were in general more advanced in social development and had higher IQs. No evidence of harm could be found and we were able to conclude that joint admission is a safe and useful procedure. In addition, we were impressed at how important the nature of the participation of the father was both to the success of joint admissions and often to the effectiveness of the hospitalization of the mother. Our studies of joint admission have been published in a book, *Mentally Ill Mothers and Their Children* (Grunebaum et al., 1975b).

While these studies were being carried out, the nature of psychiatric hospitalization was changing—it was becoming shorter. Increasingly, as soon as a woman became well enough to consider a joint admission, she was discharged to the community. It became apparent, therefore, that if we were to influence for the better the parenting that children of psychotic mothers were receiving, we would have to undertake preventive intervention in the community since this was where our patients were.

With the aid of a grant from the Division of Applied Research, National Institute of Mental Health, home visits by specially trained psychiatric nurses were provided for 50 psychotic mothers who had at least one child age five and under, who were recruited from the state mental hospitals in and around the Boston area, and who volunteered to participate. The intervention was offered for either one or two years. In order to provide a relatively stringent test of the effects of treatment, we designed the study to include three groups of mothers. Two groups of 25 were formed by random assignment of the psychotic mothers. One of these groups received intensive long-term nursing aftercare while the other group received minimal contact. A third group of mothers with no psychiatric history, obtained through advertisement in local papers, was individually matched to the mothers in the other two groups on social class, ethnicity, parity, and age and sex of the youngest child. These mothers did not receive the intervention. In all instances, psychiatric home-nursing aftercare was not in lieu of, but rather in addition to, other services the families were receiving. The intervention consisted of weekly home visits lasting between 1 and 1½ hours and focused on the mother's relationship with her youngest child in particular. Since the mother was seen in her home, her interactions with her children could be directly observed and discussed. The effects of the psychotic experience and unresolved issues in the mother's own life were also important subjects. While the two high-risk groups did not differ in other treatment parameters such as the use of drugs or other treatment, the intensive treatment group received 1384 home visits while the minimally treated group was visited 130 times.

At the time of admission to the study and at termination of the intervention a series of assessments of the mother and her youngest child were made. These included, for the mother: the Minnesota Multiphasic Personality Inventory (MMPI), a social-role performance evaluation interview, and a clinical interview of both the mother and her husband when he was willing. The child was administered an age-appropriate intelligence test. Ratings were made of the child's behavior, affect, and social interactions during the testing. Child psychiatric evaluations were also carried out.

Let us turn to the mothers' findings first. The two treatment groups turned out to be well matched. The majority of the women were lower middle-class, in their late 20s, chronically psychotic, usually diagnosed schizophrenic, and functioning rather poorly. Comparisons were made of the findings at the time of termination and there were no significant differences between the groups in diagnosis, chronicity, or duration of hospitalization. The results of the intervention are rather striking (self-report differing from objective measures). The intensive treatment group reported greater feelings of self-worth and a sense of having been helped than did the group that received only minimal aftercare. However, this finding is at variance with the results of the MMPI, the evaluation of social-role performance, the frequency of rehospitalization, and the reports of their husbands at the time of termination. It is clear that the assistance of the nurse was experienced by the mothers as helpful in specific areas, but there are no objective data to support this view. In part, differences between the groups may have been minimized by virtue of the fact that the nurse was always potentially available to the minimally treated groups; in times of crisis, phone contacts were frequent and referrals to other agencies were often made. For ethical reasons one cannot permit families to founder.

Investigation of about 30 fathers was less complete and we were only able to rate their role in the family, their health, and their work history. About one-half of the fathers were actively involved with their wives and in parenting their children. The other half were as impaired as the mothers. They were either unable to work or were alcoholics. It is of note that not a single child who had an inadequately functioning father was rated as functioning even moderately well at termination of the study, while children of adequate fathers ranged from moderately poor to good in their functioning.

Let us now turn to the evaluation of the effects of this program on the children. There were no significant differences in intellectual performance between the two groups. Affectively, however, the children from the intensive treatment group were less inhibited, less withdrawn, less anxious, and less negative. They had less difficulty with task performance and required less help from the examiner. Compared with the minimally treated group, they were more involved with people than things, but this finding may be due to a small group of severely inhibited children in the minimally treated group. There were no differences in IQ level, or IQ variability, or observed maternal behavior in the testing situation. The evaluation of the child psychiatrist did differ in the two groups. To the degree that these findings cannot be attributed to examiner bias, we can conclude that the intensive intervention program did have a favorable influence on the children's development.

Why did the intervention appear to have some impact on the children and none on their mothers? Two possibilities may be suggested. First, it is likely that the mothers, many of whom suffered from long-standing chronic problems of adaptation and psychological distress, were less amenable to change than the children. Second, it may be that effects on the children of periods of crisis and distress, although equally frequent in the two groups, were buffered in the intensively treated group. Finally, it may be that the objective assessments of the mother were insufficiently sensitive to pick up changes in her which she was aware of, such as improved morale, and which favorably influenced her child, if only slightly.

We have arrived at the following conclusions based on our five-year efforts at psychiatric intervention:

1. Generalizations about the effectiveness of therapeutic intervention for mothers based on the study should be made with great care since our research population was typically lower middle-class, largely chronic schizophrenic women and their children. Probably, the better adjusted and better educated the mother, the greater will be the impact of psychiatric intervention.

2. Increasingly, we have come to believe that the children of psychotic mothers should be offered psychiatric assistance on a continuing basis. Anthony (1972) has suggested some useful components of long-term intervention. It is often difficult, however, to gain access to the children or the home for such preventive efforts, particularly if the psychotic mother is paranoid or tends to deny her illness, and particularly if she is the only parent in the home. We will have to learn to accept the limitations of psychotherapy and pharmacotherapy and be prepared to provide homemakers and to arrange for foster care.

3. It may be particularly useful to offer support and counseling to the fathers if they are available. Family therapists often find work with the healthier member of the family most productive for positive change. Traditionally, the approach to the healthier spouse has been to offer support and to foster a willingness to accept the patient's idiosyncrasies. Our work suggests that the father should be mobilized to supply needed parenting to his children and should be aided in his efforts to intervene constructively in the mother's pathogenic interactions with her children rather than be a passive, helpless, or uninvolved bystander. The development of a program of preventive

intervention with fathers will demand changing our usual practice; more of the workers will have to be male and the father may well have to be seen in the evening after work.

4. In the development of preventive programs, great care must be exercised so as not to impair the ability of individuals to live their lives free from the dangers of bureaucratic interference or the social consequences of being labeled as pathological. These dangers are already being encountered in the area of genetic counseling.

More recent work of our group (Cohler et al., in press) comparing children of schizophrenic and depressed mothers led to the unexpected conclusion that the children of depressed mothers are more impaired than the children of schizophrenic mothers. Children of depressed mothers show the greatest impairment in intellectual ability, particularly on tasks that involve separating figure from ground as in the embedded figures test. We are in the process of completing a five-year follow-up study that seems to confirm these results both on objective test measures and in clinical interviews (Grunebaum et al., 1976, unpublished data). The results of this follow-up study suggest that the most creative and successful of the children of psychotic parents we have studied have schizophrenic mothers, while the most impaired have depressed mothers. This is in accord with other studies such as those of Karlsson (1966) and that of Heston and Denney (1968).

In view of these findings and based on our experience, we currently plan to locate *all* children who have psychotic mothers in Cambridge-Somerville, the catchment area for which we are responsible. We will attempt to provide each family with a contact person on the staff who will keep in touch with them and whom they may call in time of need. It is not our expectation that the contact person should, or could, be the family's sole therapist—for no one can deal adequately with adults and children, psychotherapy and drugs, community resources and psychodynamics. Rather, the family members should have someone to turn to when they need help and someone who keeps track of them. For these seriously troubled families, a family mental health general practitioner who can evaluate the problems, make referrals, and act as an ombudsman for the family in the mental health system is indicated, for multiproblem families such as these tend to receive care that is fragmented in terms of agencies, caregivers, focus, and time. Since the problems are likely to last for many years, the approach should be one of long-term contact and periodic intervention during crises only.

The focus of work that this contact person could provide has been discussed by David Ricks in his remarkable paper, "Supershrink: Methods of a Therapist Judged Successful on the Basis of Adult Outcomes of Adolescent Patients" (Ricks, 1972). Although this study is not usually considered in the discussion of high-risk populations and primary prevention of psychosis, it contains observations of great importance to the conduct of therapy and for teachers of therapists.

As an outgrowth of Ricks' investigation of children who were first seen in a child guidance clinic in Boston and who became schizophrenic as adults, he compared the therapeutic success of two therapists who had treated comparable numbers of disturbed children. The comparison was based on adult outcomes as measured by the number of patients who became schizophrenic as adults, and in terms of social functioning. One of the therapists, nicknamed "Supershrink" by the children, had only four of the 15 patients whom he had seen as children develop schizophrenia as adults. The "unsuccessful" therapist had as patients 13 children who became schizophrenic in adulthood; three of them became chronic schizophrenics. The social functioning of the two groups of patients in adulthood was also markedly different. "Supershrink's" patients had a much more adequate level of social functioning.

Ricks studied the records of the two therapists as far back as possible. Both therapists had begun with very similar caseloads (all the patients were boys). The cases were also similar on demographic variables and, most importantly, on severity of pathology at the time they were first seen.

How, then, did these two therapists differ? First of all, it is important to note that "Supershrink" spent far more time with the children who were most disturbed while the other therapist allocated more time to the healthier children. In addition, the "unsuccessful" therapist seemed to become discouraged by the vulnerability of some of his patients and tended to focus his attention on the child's anxiety and depressive feelings, thus overloading an already tenuous therapeutic relationship. A second difference was that the unsuccessful therapist was exceedingly active in his use of resources outside the immediate treatment situation such as camps, foster homes, and boarding schools. He was noteworthy in the thoroughness and care with which he helped the boys work out these arrangements. "Supershrink" was firm, active, and direct in his relationship with the children's parents, meeting with them frequently in an era when this approach was unusual. Central to this family-interaction approach was his support of the boys in their efforts toward autonomy.

Finally, there was a difference, which, as Rick states, ". . . begins in a seemingly trivial observation and ends in a mystery." It is that "Supershrink's" files contained many letters from the "boys," some written many years later, and his notes of the many spontaneous visits they made to the clinic to visit him. It seems that he had become an anchor in reality (a friend) to these boys. Ricks reviewed "Supershrink's" therapy notes and believes that the following were critical to this therapeutic success: First, every therapy hour had to be useful, and if it was not he wanted to know why; second, he was unusually open to the boys' feelings, was direct and open about his own feelings, and was unthreatened by the boys' feelings. The other therapist tended to be distant, cognitive, and interested particularly in feelings of depression and anxiety rather than in the entire scope of the boys' lives. Finally, "Supershrink" actively promoted his patients' competence in handling their own problems; by the devices of example and modeling he often expressed his own opinions on how alternative ways of problem-solving might be looked at, and on the consequences of different courses of action.

I have taken some time to review this beautifully written and carefully thought-out study by Ricks because it illustrates all too painfully that clinicians are not cognizant of the extent of their own influence on patient outcome. Such conclusions are often hidden in the mass of data on the outcome of psychotherapy, but the finding that therapists can be harmful as well as helpful is increasingly clear, as Bergin (1971) demonstrates in his review of the literature.

Having suggested that our attitudes and behavior as mental health professionals influence our efforts at prevention, I should like to conclude this journey by suggesting that it is the fact that we *are* mental health professionals that prevents us from incorporating into our work settings the simplest, cheapest, most effective, and most direct forms of prevention. Given the pressures of clinical practice and the priorities of our profession, we do not actively seek to promote responsible fertility with our patients. At this point, I should like to sell you on the idea that family-planning counseling and contraceptive services should be a prime task of mental health professionals who work with families under the stress of mental illness. Research has shown that mentally ill women have a large number of unplanned and unwanted pregnancies and their children are likely to be at risk for psychological, social, and educational impairment (Abernethy and Grunebaum, 1972; Abernethy, 1973; Abernethy et al., 1975; Grunebaum et al., 1971; Grunebaum and Abernethy, 1974, 1975; Grunebaum et al., 1975a).

Additional births are a stress to an already burdened woman and her family and may lead to a recurrence of her illness. With the widespread therapeutic use of psychotropic drugs that render the patient socially functional, and because of partial hospitalizations and increased sexual freedom, we are faced with an increasing birth rate among the mentally ill. A 12-percent increase in the birth rate was found by Erlenmeyer-Kimling (in press) between 1934-1936 and 1954-1956, and we suspect that this trend has continued. In addition, the mentally ill population has special difficulties in making informed and balanced decisions about sexual behavior and fertility since many patients are only at marginal functional levels. Many are impulsive and immature adolescents, and recent work suggests that these are an increasing proportion of the psychotic mothers of young children. Referral to community-based family-planning clinics is rarely successful; therefore, family-planning counseling should be an integral part of treatment.

Our studies demonstrate that psychiatric patients desire contraceptive assistance, but it is rarely suggested by mental health professionals and it is certainly not a routine part of treatment planning. However, when family-planning counseling and services are provided in the mental hospital, they are welcomed and used; with ongoing support from the counselor, continuation rates after discharge are excellent. What resistance there is comes from the staff, not the patients. With the aid of a grant, initially from the Office of Economic Opportunity and now from the Office of Family Planning, we have counseled and provided contraception for more than 1000 women in three state mental hospitals in Massachusetts in the last three years. In this day of rapid discharges, short-term hospitalization, and community-based care, helping a woman to plan her family should be part of total care. It is, in addition, a safe and effective form of prevention.

What are we to conclude from this foray into the area of research on individuals at high risk of becoming psychotic? In thinking about preventive intervention, it is useful to remember first that most healthy people will not thank us for interfering with their lives. It would be most upsetting to be told that one had a fairly good chance of ending up "crazy" if there were nothing one could do about it in the meanwhile, in spite of the fact that it seems evident that the odds that a given person will become psychotic and the likelihood that this outcome can be prevented are important to know.

We have discussed two significant groups of children who may be vulnerable to schizophrenia or other forms of psychopathology. One group consists of shy and friendless girls, and obstreperous and friendless boys, particularly if their difficulties increase as they become adolescent. These are children who actively avoid other children and whose acting-out is inappropriate rather than part of normal peer-group interaction. Fortunately, these children are the ones that child guidance counselors are likely to see, and schools should be encouraged to refer these children for counseling.

The second group is made up of the children of psychotic mothers. It seems evident that we should try to develop services so that families of a psychotic parent receive special attention and that we seek them out rather than vice versa. As I have suggested, some sort of a family mental health worker who would act as an ombudsman for the family with the various agencies and resources within the community would be most valuable. This person would keep in touch with the family and keep track of them and their problems. He/she would deal with them realistically and would strive to foster competence and coping. The duration of these efforts should be long and the focus should be on the promotion of competence, toward which the use of community resources will be a major component.

Finally, I have suggested that probably the cheapest, most effective, and surest prevention measure currently available is voluntary contraceptive services for the mentally ill.

Even if we were to undertake all the measures that I have outlined, however, it is not at all certain that we would significantly reduce the number of psychotics. Perhaps we will only have a positive influence on the level of milder psychopathology, and perhaps not even that. I should like to offer some comfort and solace by reminding you of Manfred Bleuler's studies (1974) of children who grew up in homes with a psychotic parent, and his eloquent comments as to the tragedy of that experience: "In short, the sufferings that the children endure can continue to affect their lives even when they do not interfere with their health or professional attainment. Any horrible experience remembered from childhood can continue to hurt and to cast its shadow over life's happiness." Perhaps some of our clinical efforts may at least mitigate human tragedy as we accompany families through it.

REFERENCES

ABERNETHY, V., 1973. Family planning in two psychiatric hospitals: A preliminary report. *Fam. Plann. Perspect.* 5 (2):94-99.
ABERNETHY, V., and GRUNEBAUM, H. 1972. Toward a family planning program in psychiatric hospitals. *Am. J. Public Health,* 62 (12):1638-1646.
ABERNETHY, V., ROBBINS, D., ABERNETHY, G., GRUNEBAUM, H., and WEISS, J. 1975. Identification of women at risk for unwanted pregnancy. *Am. J. Public Health,* 132:10.
ANTHONY, E. J. 1968. The developmental precursors of adult schizophrenia. In D. Rosenthal and S. S. Kety (eds.), *The Transmission of Schizophrenia,* pp. 293-316. Elmsford, N.Y.: Pergamon Press.
ANTHONY, E. J. 1969. A clinical evaluation of children with psychotic parents. *Am. J. Psychiatry,* 126 (2):177-184.

ANTHONY, E. J. 1970. The impact of mental and physical illness on family life. *Am. J. Psychiatry*, 127:138-146.

ANTHONY, E. J. 1972. Primary prevention with school children. In H. H. Barten and L. Bellak (eds.), *Progress in Community Mental Health*, vol. 2, pp. 131-158. New York: Grune & Stratton.

BERGIN, A. E., 1971. The evaluation of therapeutic outcomes. In A. E. Bergin and S. I. Garfield (eds.), *Handbook of Psychotherapy and Behavior Change*. New York: Wiley.

BLEULER, M. 1974. The offspring of schizophrenics. *Schizophrenia Bulletin*, 8:93-109.

COHLER, B., WEISS, J., WOOLSEY, S., and GRUNEBAUM, H. 1968. Childrearing attitudes among mothers volunteering and revolunteering for a psychological study. *Psychol. Rep.*, 23:603-612.

COHLER, B., WEISS, J., and GRUNEBAUM, H. 1970. Childcare attitudes and emotional disturbances among mothers of young children. *Genet. Psychol. Monogr.*, 82:3-47.

COHLER, B., GRUNEBAUM, H., WEISS, J., GAMER, E., and GALLANT, D. Disturbance of attention among schizophrenic, depressed and well mothers and their young children. *J. Child Psychol. Psychiatry*, in press.

ERLENMEYER-KIMLING, L. Fertilité des psychotiques. Démographie. *Confrontations Psychiatriques*, in press.

GAMER, E., and GRUNEBAUM, H. 1976. Children of psychotic mothers: An evaluation of 1-year olds on a test of object permanence. *Arch. Gen. Psychiatry*, 33:311-317.

GAMER, E., GRUNEBAUM, H., COHLER, B., and GALLANT, D. Children at risk: Performance of 3-year olds and their mentally ill and well mothers on interaction tasks. Unpublished manuscript.

GARMEZY, N. 1974a. Children at risk: The search for the antecedents of schizophrenia. Part I. Conceptual modes and research methods. *Schizophrenia Bulletin*, 8:14-91.

GARMEZY, N. 1974b. Children at risk: The search for the antecedents of schizophrenia. Part II. Ongoing research programs, issues, and intervention. *Schizophrenia Bulletin*, 9:55-126.

GARMEZY, N. 1975. Review of current knowledge of early detection: Characteristics of high-risk subjects. Meeting of the Working Group on Primary Prevention of Schizophrenia in High-Risk Groups, Copenhagen.

GOLDSTEIN, M. J. 1975. Psychotherapeutic intervention with families of adolescents at risk for schizophrenia. Meeting of the Working Group on Primary Prevention of Schizophrenia in High-Risk Groups, Copenhagen.

GOLDSTEIN, M. J., JUDD, L. L., RODNICK, E. H., ALKIRE, A., and GOULD, E. A. 1968. A method for studying social influence and coping patterns within families of disturbed adolescents. *J. Nerv. Ment. Dis.*, 147 (3):233-251.

GRUNEBAUM, H., GALLANT, D., COHLER, B., KAUFFMAN, C., and GAMER, E. 1976. Children of psychotic mothers: A five-year follow-up study. Unpublished data.

GRUNEBAUM, H. 1975. Preventive intervention with psychotic mothers: A controlled study. Meeting of the Working Group on Primary Prevention of Schizophrenia in High-Risk Groups, Copenhagen.

GRUNEBAUM, H., and ABERNETHY, V. 1974. Marital decision making as applied to family planning. *Journal of Sex and Marital Therapy*, 1 (1):63-74.

GRUNEBAUM, H., and ABERNETHY, V. 1975. Ethical issues in family planning for hospitalized psychiatric patients. *Am. J. Psychiatry*, 132:33, 236-240.

GRUNEBAUM, H., ABERNETHY, V., ROFMAN, S., and WEISS, J. 1971. Family planning attitudes, practices and motivations of mental patients. *Am. J. Psychiatry*, 128:6.

GRUNEBAUM, H., WEISS, J., GALLANT, D., HARTMAN, C., GAMER, E., and ABERNETHY, V. 1974. Attention in young children of psychotic mothers. *Am. J. Psychiatry*, 131:8.

GRUNEBAUM, H., ABERNETHY, V., CLOUGH, L., and GROOVER, B. 1975a. Staff attitudes toward a family planning service in the mental hospital. *Community Ment. Health J.,* 2 (3):280-285.

Grunebaum, H., Weiss, J., Cohler, B., Gallant, D., and Hartman, C. 1975b. *Mentally Ill Mothers and Their Children.* Chicago: University of Chicago Press.

Heston, L. L., and Denney, D. 1968. Interactions between early life experience and biological factors in schizophrenia. In D. Rosenthal and S. S. Kety (eds.), *The Transmission of Schizophrenia,* pp. 363-376. Elmsford, N.Y.: Pergamon Press.

Karlsson, J. 1966. *The Biological Basis for Schizophrenia.* Springfield, Ill.: Thomas.

Ricks, D. F. 1972. Supershrink: Methods of a therapist judged successful on the basis of adult outcomes of adolescent patients. In M. Roff and D. E. Ricks (eds.), *Life History Research in Psychopathology.* Minneapolis: University of Minnesota Press.

Rodnick, E. H., and Goldstein, M. J. 1972. A research strategy for studying risk for schizophrenia during adolescence and early adulthood. Presented at Conference on Risk Research, Dorado Beach, Puerto Rico.

Rolf, J. E. 1972. The academic and social competence of children vulnerable to schizophrenia and other behavior pathologies. *J. Abnorm. Psychol.,* 80 (3):225-243.

Rolf, J. E., and Garmezy, N. The school performance of children vulnerable to behavior pathology. In D. F. Ricks, A. Thomas, and M. Roff (eds.), *Life History Research in Psychopathology,* vol. 3. Minneapolis: University of Minnesota Press, in press.

Rolf, J. E., and Harig, P. T. 1974. Etiological research in schizophrenia and the rationale of primary interventions. *Am. J. Orthopsychiatry,* 44 (4):538-557.

Watt, N. F. 1972. Longitudinal changes in the social behavior of children hospitalized for schizophrenia as adults. *Am. J. Orthopsychiatry,* 40 (4):637-657.

Watt, N. F. 1976. Research bases for change in clinical practice: I. The longitudinal base for early intervention. Paper read at the Society for Psychotherapy Research. Unpublished.

Watt, N. F. Childhood roots of schizophrenia. In D. F. Ricks, A. Thomas, and M. Roff (eds.), *Life History Research in Psychopathology,* vol. 3. Minneapolis: University of Minnesota Press, in press.

Watt, N. F., Stolorow, R. D., Lubensky, A. W., and McClelland, D. C. 1970. School adjustment and behavior of children hospitalized for schizophrenia as adults. *Am. J. Orthopsychiatry,* 40:637-657.

Wynne, L. C. Emerging trends in family research on schizophrenia. In M. M. Katz, R. Littlestone, L. R. Mosher, A. Tuma, and M. Roath (eds.), *Schizophrenia: Implications of Research Findings for Treatment and Teaching,* in press.

Wynne, L. C. 1967. Family transactions and schizophrenia. II: Conceptual considerations for a research strategy. In J. Romano (ed.), *The Origins of Schizophrenia,* pp. 165-178. Amsterdam: Excerpta Medica Foundation.

Wynne, L. C. 1968. Methodologic and conceptual issues in the study of schizophrenics and their families. In D. Rosenthal and S. S. Kety (eds.), *The Transmission of Schizophrenia,* pp. 185-199. Elmsford, N.Y.: Pergamon Press.

Wynne, L. C., and Singer, M. T. 1963. Thought disorder and family relations of schizophrenics: A research strategy. *Arch. Gen. Psychiatry,* 9:191-198.

11

Family Structure and Interaction: Sibling Effects on Socialization

VICTOR G. CICIRELLI, Ph.D.

Over the past several years, there has been a steadily increasing emphasis on family therapy in child psychiatry and child clinical psychology. This is based on the view of the family as a dynamic system in which a change in one family member affects all other family members. The family system, however, tends to be stable and resistant to change (Handel, 1965) when one member is engaged in therapy. To bring about desired changes, one must therefore work with the entire family system, and to do so one needs to understand how the family system operates to influence its members.

Family members socialize each other as they perceive, communicate, interact, and coordinate their behaviors with each other so that both the family as a unit and individual members can adapt and develop over the life span. Although family members socialize each other in a reciprocal manner, parents and older children have greater influence on younger children than vice versa, since they have greater maturity and power within the family.

The way that family members communicate and interact with each other depends on the family structure. By family structure is meant a network of positions defined by age, sex, and age difference for the parents, and by birth order, age, sex, and age difference for the children. Each position involves roles relative to other positions in the network as determined by cultural norms and values. A mother, for example, enacts certain roles and holds certain role expectations regarding the father, and a different set of behaviors and expectations regarding a first-born son.

In short, family structure influences the manner of interaction between family members, and the resulting socialization leads to changes in characteristics of both the family as a unit and individual family members as the family system adapts and grows in response to new and changing environmental conditions.

The family can be viewed as an interactional network consisting of three subsystems: parent-parent interactions, parent-child interactions, and sibling-sibling interactions. (As a more general formulation for families including extended family members, adopted children, half-siblings, and so on, one can speak of adult-adult interactions, adult-child interactions, and child-child interactions.) For each subsystem, interactions between the family members concerned involve certain patterns and mutual experiences that distinguish them from other subsystems. Thus, one can look at a particular subsystem as partially independent of the family as a whole.

Much research has been done to show how parents interact with each other and how parents socialize their children. Particular attention has been paid to the mother-child relationship. The sibling-sibling subsystem, in contrast, has been almost ignored.

It is the thesis of this paper that siblings are important agents of family socialization in two ways: (1) They aid in socializing each other throughout the life span; they directly influence each other. (2) Siblings influence each other indirectly, through their effect on parent-parent and parent-child interactions.

My research has provided some evidence for these statements, at least in regard to the influence of a child's siblings on such aspects of cognitive development as concept formation, problem solving, and cognitive styles. Before discussing the results of these studies, however, I would like to consider some of the general characteristics of sibling-sibling interactions.

Siblings Socialize Each Other

According to sociologist Donald P. Irish (1964), bonds between siblings extend throughout life and are second only to mother-child ties. He sees siblings as fulfilling a number of functions: parent substitutes, teachers of youthful skills, role models, challengers, and stimulators.

Within the family, siblings may influence each other to a greater extent than parents under certain conditions and for certain tasks. Young children can learn certain tasks more effectively if they are taught by a person closer to their age (who understands their problems and viewpoint and can communicate at the same language level) than by a parent. This may be especially true for certain tasks (school activities, youthful skills, dealing with difficult teachers, bullies, and so on), taboo subjects (sex, drugs, revolutionary ideas, death), and for certain personal-social characteristics (sex-role identity, appearance, and behavior) in which parents and other adults are unwilling or incapable of helping children. Older siblings may be more effective teachers for these tasks.

If one considers the siblings (at least those relatively close in age) as a peer group, then the "family peer group" can be compared with the nonfamily peer group (Cicirelli, 1976c). There are many similarities between the family and nonfamily peer-group systems. Activities that occur in the peer group are also likely to occur in a family peer group of equal size and age level. In both cases peers can be models, reinforcers, caretakers, confidants, and pacesetters, as well as teachers.

There are several differences, however, between family and nonfamily peers. First, there is a greater amount of interaction, or more frequently repeated interaction between family peers than nonfamily peers. The sibling relationship is one of extensive intimate daily contact; thus a sibling pair establishes a pattern of communication and responsiveness to each other. One aspect of this interaction pattern is an educative function in which information is transmitted from one sibling to another, gradually shaping abilities and styles of learning. Second, the group structure or association between family peer members is more durable than a voluntary association of nonfamily peers (e.g., a child may have a "falling out" with a friend and the relationship may be ended. But if a child has a "falling out" with a sibling, they must "patch things up" and continue the relationship). Third, ascribed (nonchosen) roles exist in a family peer group along with achieved (chosen) roles so that a child is accepted by virtue of his family membership rather than for what he does. Fourth, there is greater commonality in the family peer group since all family peer members are socialized by the same two dominant members of the family interaction system, the parents. Thus siblings are likely to share common values and attitudes which facilitate the influence of sibs on each other. These differences between the family peer group and the nonfamily peer group mean that there is greater-opportunity for family peers to provide empathy, rapport, and communication. In sum, family peers have greater opportunity for socializing a family member than do nonfamily peers.

Important also are the long-range advantages of sibling relationships. As siblings interact and teach and help each other from day to day, they develop caring relationships and will turn to each other for help when needed. Research has shown that siblings maintain fairly frequent contact throughout life (Adams, 1968); indeed, Cumming and Schneider (1961) report that the bond between sisters may be even stronger than a bond to the spouse in old age. Adams (1968) found that rivalry and comparison between brothers remained important in adulthood, thus indicating that family-interaction patterns formed early in life remain in later years. A recent study of mine (Cicirelli, 1977b) revealed that the older person's siblings provided important emotional support as they faced common problems of aging.

Effects of Sibling Structure

The bulk of sibling research done so far has attempted to demonstrate that certain characteristics of a child are related to that child's position in the sibling structure. (The sibling structure of a family is the network of positions of children in the family defined by the number of children, birth order, sex of the children, their ages, and the age spacing between them. A given child's sibling status in relation to the sibling structure is his/her position in that network.)

Different investigators have emphasized particular aspects of the sibling structure. Some have considered only birth order and/or family size for children of a given age while ignoring the effects of age spacing and sex. Anastasi (1956) summarized much of the early work in this area, which indicated that larger family size and a later birth order were associated with poorer cognitive ability and performance, although such effects were diminished or absent at higher socioeconomic levels. More recent work includes the critical arguments of Schooler (1972), the studies of Belmont and Marolla (1973), and those of Zajonc and Markus (1975).

Another line of research has considered the effects of sex of the child and siblings, and age spacing, while holding age, family size, and birth order constant or considering them only in a limited way. Helen Koch's (1954) work was a pioneering effort in this field. Results of these studies are too detailed to summarize here; the reader is referred to the work of Sutton-Smith and Rosenberg (1970).

Sibling structure effects on cognitive styles have had little investigation. Among college students, Stewart (1967) found first-born males to be more field-dependent than last-born males; Eisenman (1967) found first-born males and later-born females to prefer greater stimulus complexity than later-born males and first-born females. With kindergarten children, Koch (1954) found that second-born children exceeded first-born children on tests of perceptual speed; among those separated by a wide age spacing, there was a tendency for those with a brother to have greater perceptual speed than those with a sister. Finally, Bigner (1974) found that second-born elementary school children described female siblings less abstractly than male siblings, and they also described older siblings who were close in age less abstractly than older siblings who were more widely spaced.

A variety of explanations has been proposed for the apparent effects of the sibling-structure variables. One explanation (e.g., Rothbart, 1976) is that the parent treats the child differently, depending on sex and birth order. Role theory provides another possible explanation (Bossard and Boll, 1960); for example, older sisters are more likely to be delegated caretaking or teaching roles in the family. These explanations deal with the influence of the parent or of social norms on the child. Another group of explanatory factors deals with the influence of the siblings on each other. Sibling rivalry (Koch, 1960; Rosenberg and Sutton-Smith, 1969) that results from sibling displacement is considered to be most intense between brothers and between children two to four years apart in age. Sutton-Smith and Rosenberg (1969) proposed that modeling after certain sibling behaviors and reactivity to other behaviors may affect outcomes. Social facilitation (Cottrell, 1968) and social reinforcement (Stevenson, 1965) may also be factors in sibling-structure effects. No single explanation accounts for the findings, although each applies to a portion of the results.

Effects of Sibling Interaction

Except for certain animal studies (e.g., Harlow, 1969) and interviews of siblings by Sutton-Smith and Rosenberg (1970), direct studies of the interaction between siblings and its effect on sibling outcome had not been done when I began a series of studies five years ago (Cicirelli, 1972; 1973; 1974; 1975; 1976a, b, c, d; 1977a).

The studies involve variants of the same basic experimental paradigm. They were typical laboratory experiments carried out in the field (at school or in homes) with enough controls so that the effects could be ascribed to the experimental treatment factor. The studies involved white, primarily middle-class children in the primary grades. Age spacing was held constant at two years in most studies (although two- and four-year spacings were investigated in one study). Family size was controlled at two children or not investigated (although one study considered small and large family sizes). Birth order was not investigated; the focal child of the study was always a younger sibling (a second-born or later-born child of the family). The interaction of this child with an older sibling (a first-born or earlier-born child) was studied. Sex of the child and sex of the older sibling were considered in each study. Children from families with the desired sibling-structure characteristics were identified in the general school population and divided into four sex subgroups: boys with older brothers, boys with older sisters, girls with older brothers, and girls with older sisters. (If an additional sibling-structure variable was investigated, each of the four groups was further subdivided—into larger- and small-family subgroups, for example, or two- and four-year age spacings.) Subjects from each subgroup were randomly assigned to experimental treatment and control conditions. In the "sibling" experimental condition, the child was aided by the older sibling in practicing a cognitive task while the interaction was observed; in a subsequent test session, the child worked alone on an alternate form of the task. In the control condition, the child worked alone during the practice session. (In some of the studies, a second experimental group was used in which the mother helped the child on the practice task. One study used a comparison group of re-paired siblings in which the younger child was helped by an unrelated older child who had the same sibling status as the younger child's own sibling.)

Two kinds of data come out of such a study: observational measures of the interaction between the younger child and the older helper on the practice task, and measures of the younger child's performance on the test version of the task. Thus the effect of sibling-structure variables and of the experimental conditions can be determined in relation to both the sibling-interaction process and the task outcome (as well as the relationships between the process and outcome measures).

This experimental paradigm is based on the assumption that what occurs in the experimental situation represents sibling interactions that occur in the home when cognitive tasks (schoolwork, games, etc.) are done. If interactions between siblings take on enduring, characteristic patterns, then these patterns should appear in the experimental situation as well as at home. If this is true, then influence of older siblings on younger ones in the laboratory situation may be interpreted as evidence of socialization.

The first study (Cicirelli, 1972) investigated sibling interaction as the older child taught a concept (a trapezoid) to the younger child. For half of 120 children, the older sibling was the teacher; for the remaining half, siblings were re-paired so that the child was taught by a nonsibling. The older child was trained in the concept to a given learning criterion in a standardized teaching session that involved several teaching techniques. Then the older child was asked to teach the concept to the younger one in a 10-minute session, after which the younger child was given a concept-attainment test. Older sisters were found to be significantly more effective teachers of younger siblings than older girls were of unrelated younger children, while older boys were more effective teachers of unrelated younger children than of their own younger siblings. Viewed in another way, older sisters were significantly more effective teachers of younger siblings than were older brothers. Older boys and girls were not significantly different in effectiveness as teachers of nonsiblings, even though these unrelated children occupied the same sibling status positions as the older children's own siblings. Girls teaching their younger siblings used a deductive teaching method (explaining and describing, demonstrating and illustrating attributes of the concept), while boys teaching their siblings used an inductive approach (presenting many examples and allowing the learner to abstract the concept himself).

Another study (Cicirelli, 1975, 1976b) used a problem-solving task in which the younger child was aided in determining which of alternative patterns was the correct one (i.e., lights in a pre-set 5 x 5 matrix of bulbs would go on to form this pattern when pressed) by the older sibling or by the mother. A control group worked on the problems alone in the practice session. Half of the 120 subjects were from two-child families and half from larger families. Children with older brothers performed as well alone as after aid by their brother or mother, while children with older sisters showed more advanced problem-solving after being helped by their sister or mother. Children with the same-sex siblings completed the problems more rapidly than children with opposite-sex siblings. Family size had no effect. When the family interaction patterns were examined, it was found that older sisters gave more explanation, more feedback, and more total verbalization about the task than did older brothers. Mothers, however, gave more explanation and feedback and more total verbalization to children with older brothers than to children with older sisters. This suggests that the mother relinquishes a portion of her helping role toward a child when that child has an older sister. It was also found that children from large families sought and were given more help on the task than children from small families; both mothers and older siblings displayed more explanatory behaviors and more total verbalization, tending to tell the child just what moves to make in solving the problem and even to tell him or her the correct answer to it.

The two studies established two important points. The first was that siblings do affect each other directly, with a sibling pair both teaching and learning differently when interacting with each other than when interacting with a nonsibling. If only parent influences due to sibling structure were acting, one would expect the children to behave the same in both situations. Second, there is an indirect effect of sibling-sibling interactions on the mother-child interactions. Receptiveness to help from older sisters and independence regarding help from older brothers are well-establishd characteristics that transfer to a situation in which the sibling is absent and the mother is offering help.

Two studies have determined the influence of siblings on the child's cognitive styles. An object-sorting task (Wallach and Kogan, 1970) , in which the child was asked to sort 50 pictures of common objects into groups of his choice, was used to obtain measures of categorization and conceptual styles. Categorization style includes conceptual differentiation (number of groups formed), compartmentalization (number of objects left ungrouped) , and "bandwidth" (number of objects in a group) . Conceptual style refers to the logical basis for grouping objects together. A child who uses descriptive-analytic groupings bases them on similarity between objective physical attributes among a group of objects; in categorical-inferential groupings, a child bases the selection on the objects' shared characteristic so that each object is an example of the superordinate concept; relational-thematic groupings are based on a functional or thematic relationship between the objects in a group.

The first of these studies (Cicirelli, 1973, 1974) varied both age of the child and age spacing between siblings in two-child families; half the children were of kindergarten age and half were in the second grade; their older siblings were either two or four years older.

Half of the 160 subjects were helped by their sibling on a practice object-sorting task, and the rest worked alone. We found that children who had been helped by their sibling in the practice task made more groups and left fewer objects ungrouped than did children who had worked alone. The effect was greatest when the sibling was four years older. Use of descriptive-analytic categories, which typically declines with age (Cicirelli, 1976a), was lower among children who had been helped by siblings, particularly kindergarten-age children. The use of categorical-inferential groupings was also influenced by the older sibling, but it depended on both sex and age spacing in a complex way. Use of relational-thematic categories was not affected. In the helping session, the older sibling was more likely to give cues and hints for grouping when the younger sibling was a girl. Older sisters were more likely to point to objects for grouping and to add to the child's groups than were older brothers. The younger child was more likely to accept direction and help on the task when the older sibling was a girl or four years older and was more likely to work independently on the task when the older sibling was a boy or only two years older.

The most recent study (Cicirelli, 1977a) considered family size in addition to sex of the children and compared children who had been aided by the older sibling, children who had been aided by the mother, and children who had worked alone on a practice object-sorting task preparatory to their subsequent object-sorting performance. Subjects were 120 first-grade children. Only the results for the conceptual-style measures are available thus far. Children who had been helped by their sibling or mother used fewer descriptive categories and more inferential categories than did children who had worked alone. Children helped by older sisters used more inferential categories and more descriptive categories than did children helped by older brothers. When children were helped by the mother, those with older brothers used fewer inferential categories and fewer descriptive categories than did children who had older sisters. Fewer descriptive categories were used by children from small families than by those from large families. The results of this study are not completely consistent with those of the earlier studies, but they again indicate the effects of the sibling-sibling interaction on the mother-child interaction.

SOME CONCLUSIONS AND HYPOTHESES

The results of the studies on sibling influences are more complex than can be communicated in a brief overview. One must remember also that these studies dealt with the cognitive realm, and involved primarily white, middle-class, primary-grade children from two-child families. Taken as a whole, however, the results indicate that older siblings are important socializing agents in the family. More specifically:

1. Under certain conditions and for certain tasks, older siblings are as effective as parents in helping younger siblings, and more effective than nonsiblings.

2. Within the family, the older sibling from certain sibling dyads is a more effective helper of the younger sibling than is the case in other sibling dyads. Thus, having an older sister or a sibling at a wider age spacing seems to lead to more effective help for the younger sibling.

3. Siblings who provide effective help on cognitive tasks tend to give more explanation, demonstration, cues, hints, and feedback, while less effective sibling helpers tend to use a nondirective or laissez-faire approach. A didactic approach appears to be more effective with these young children.

4. The effect of the mother as helper to the young child on a cognitive task depends on the sibling structure of the family (sex of the children, age, age spacing) and the resulting interaction pattern between the siblings. Mothers are more effective (even though they try to help less) when the older sibling is a girl, and less effective (even though they try harder) when the older sibling is a boy. The mother and younger sibling each seem to have certain role expectations and interaction patterns regarding the older sibling, and these transfer to their interaction with each other. This facilitates the

mother's influence when the older sibling is a girl and reduces it when the older sibling is a boy.

What implications do these findings have for the psychiatrist or clinician working with the child? Obviously, one cannot make direct inferences or recommendations. But I would like to advance some hypotheses that might be explored when working with family members who have mild emotional problems, or when the goal is to prevent mental illness or foster mental health. (These hypotheses are not advanced for cases in which serious conditions, such as psychosis, are present.)

I suggest the following:

1. If one accepts the family as an interactional system in which all members affect each other, it seems important to include all children in the family therapy (and especially older brothers or sisters).

However, if one considers the subsystems of the family to be semiautonomous because of uniquely shared experiences, and if the focus of the problem (s) seems to lie in a particular subsystem, then perhaps therapy should involve a sequence of sessions involving different subsystems (as well as the family as a whole), the key factor being the appropriate scheduling of the sequence.

2. If one accepts the idea that a sibling may indirectly socialize a child by influencing the parent's behavior, then in working with the parent and child one should explore the feelings, attitudes, expectations, and behavior patterns of both the parent and child toward the sibling, and determine whether these are being transferred to their interaction with each other. Perhaps clarification of the feelings of parent and child toward the sibling will clarify their own relationship to each other.

3. It may be possible to train the older sibling, particularly an older sister (or a sibling four years older), to help the younger child with mild emotional or behavioral problems, or to facilitate the mental health of the younger child.

Older siblings and peers have been used as teachers—why not as counselors? Certainly one could help an older sibling to be more open, understanding, feeling, and caring for a younger brother or sister. In the process, the older sibling's own mental health will improve through greater understanding of self and family processes.

REFERENCES

ADAMS, B. N. 1968. *Kinship in an Urban Setting*. Chicago: Markham.

ANASTASI, A. 1956. Intelligence and family size. *Psychol. Bull.*, 53:187-209.

BELMONT, L., and MAROLLA, F. A. 1973. Birth order, family size, and intelligence. *Science*, 182:1096-1101.

BIGNER, J. J. 1974. A Wernerian developmental analysis of children's descriptions of siblings. *Child Dev.*, 45:317-323.

BOSSARD, J. H. S., and BOLL, E. H. 1960. *The Sociology of Child Development*, 3rd Ed. New York: Harper & Row.

CICIRELLI, V. G. 1972. The effect of sibling relationships on concept learning of young children taught by child teachers. *Child Dev.*, 43:282-287.

CICIRELLI, V. G. 1973. Effects of sibling structure and interaction on children's categorization style. *Developmental Psychology*, 9:132-139.

CICIRELLI, V. G. 1974. Relationship of sibling structure and interaction to younger sib's conceptual style. *J. Genet. Psychol.*, 125:37-49.

CICIRELLI, V. G. 1975. Effects of mother and older sibling on the problem-solving behavior of the younger child. *Developmental Psychology*, 11:749-756.

CICIRELLI, V. G. 1976a. Categorization behavior in aging subjects. *J. Gerontol.*, 31:676-680.

CICIRELLI, V. G. 1976b. Mother-child and sibling-sibling interactions on a problem-solving task. *Child Dev.*, 47:588-596.

CICIRELLI, V. G. 1976c. Siblings helping siblings. In V. Allen (ed.), *Children as Teachers: Theory and Research on Tutoring*. New York: Academic Press.

CICIRELLI, V. G. 1976d. Sibling influence on the development of the individual. In K. F. Riegel, and J. A. Mecham (eds.), *The Developing Individual in a Changing World*, vol. 3, *Social and Environmental Issues*. Chicago: Aldine.

CICIRELLI, V. G. 1977a. Effects of mother and older sibling on child's conceptual style. *J. Genet. Psychol.*, in press.

CICIRELLI, V. G. 1977b. Relationship of siblings to the elderly person's feelings and concerns. *J. Gerontol.*, 32:317-322.

COTTRELL, N. B. 1968. Performance in the presence of other human beings: Mere presence, audience, and affiliation effects. In E. C. Simmel, R. A. Hoppe, and G. A. Milton (eds.), *Social Facilitation and Imitative Behavior*, pp. 91-110. Rockleigh, N.J.: Allyn & Bacon.

CUMMING, E., and SCHNEIDER, D. M. 1961. Sibling solidarity: A property of American kinship. *American Anthropologist*, 63:498-507.

EISENMAN, R. 1967. Complexity-simplicity. II. Birth order and sex differences. *Psychonom. Sci.*, 8:171-172.

HANDEL, G. 1965. Psychological study of whole families. *Psychol. Bull.*, 63:19-41.

HARLOW, H. F. 1969. Age-mate or peer affectional system. In D. S. Lehrman, R. A. Hinde, and E. Shaw (eds.), *Advances in the Study of Behavior*, vol. 2, pp. 333-383. New York: Academic Press.

IRISH, D. P. 1964. Sibling interaction: A neglected aspect in family life research. *Social Forces*, 42:279-288.

KOCH, H. L. 1954. The relation of primary mental abilities in five- and six-year-olds to sex of child and characteristics of his sibling. *Child Dev.*, 25:209-223.

KOCH, H. L. 1960. The relation of certain formal attributes of siblings to attitudes held toward each other and toward their parents. *Monogr. Soc. Res. Child Dev.*, 25:1-124.

ROSENBERG, B. G., and SUTTON-SMITH, B. 1969. Sibling age spacing effects upon cognition. *Developmental Psychology*, 1:661-668.

ROTHBART, M. K. 1976. Sibling position and maternal involvement. In K. F. Riegel and J. A. Mecham (eds.), *The Developing Individual in a Changing World*, vol. 3, *Social and Environmental Issues*. Chicago: Aldine.

SCHOOLER, C. 1972. Birth order effects: Not here, not now! *Psychol. Bull.*, 78:161-175.

STEVENSON, H. W. 1965. Social reinforcement of children's behavior. In L. P. Lipsett and C. C. Spiker (eds.), *Advances in Child Development and Behavior*, vol. 2, pp. 97-126. New York: Academic Press.

STEWART, R. H. 1967. Birth order and dependence. *J. Pers. Soc. Psychol.*, 6:192-194.

SUTTON-SMITH, B., and ROSENBERG, B. G. 1969. Modeling and reactive components of sibling interaction. In J. Hill (ed.), *Child Psychology*, vol. 3, *Minnesota Symposia on Child Psychology*. Minneapolis: University of Minnesota Press.

SUTTON-SMITH, B., and ROSENBERG, B. G. 1970. *The Sibling*. New York: Holt, Rinehart and Winston.

WALLACH, M. A., and KOGAN, N. 1970. *Modes of Thinking in Young Children*. New York: Holt, Rinehart and Winston.

ZAJONC, R. B., and MARKUS, G. B. 1975. Birth order and intellectual development. *Psychol. Rev.*, 82:74-88.

Part V
SOCIALIZATION RESEARCH

12

Some Clinical Applications of Research on Parent-Child Relationships

SALLY PROVENCE, M.D.

Clinicians in the fields of child development and child psychiatry are most advanced and on relatively safe ground when responding to the situation of the individual child and his family. Child-development research and clinical sophistication can be combined to provide effective treatment for developmental and psychiatric problems of early childhood. Moreover, programs that lead to early identification of developmental disorders and that provide a range of services to meet the special needs of children and their parents make the best use of the knowledge that childhood specialists now have.

In this chapter I shall limit myself to the first three years of life and, in addition, to selected studies I have found particularly helpful in conceptualizing the development of parent-child relationships and in providing the basis for child-care advice and therapeutic intervention. In mentioning particular research studies and investigators I am aware that I will be unable to acknowledge more than a small percentage of persons who have made important contributions to the current state of knowledge in this area. These investigators come from many different professional disciplines: from clinical and developmental psychology, from psychiatry and psychoanalysis, from the social sciences, from clinical social work, clinical pediatrics and nursing, and from early childhood education. Some have focused on smaller parts of the larger question, others on the broader issues.

If one accepts the task of prescribing a therapeutic environment for infants and very young children with psychological and psycho-physiological disturbances, one must be explicit about the most important characteristics of that environment. Such an environment for a young child is likely to include a number of things I have written about elsewhere (1967, 1968, 1972) but will mention briefly here. They are general enough to be considered noncontroversial, I believe, by most childhood specialists.

1. First and foremost is good physical care from a nurturing person or persons who can also provide affectionate care in accordance with the child's developmental needs. Continuity of affectionate care and the formation of close relationships with one or at most a small number of adults are still considered by many of us to be a necessary precondition for encouraging the child's development and reducing the risk of a psychiatric disturbance.

2. The child needs a speaking social partner.

3. Also needed are opportunities to *act* upon the environment, that is, to use emerging skills in a supportive and safe atmosphere.

4. Consistency and repetition in the child's experience are desirable, especially in the behavior of his caregivers so that he finds them predictable and supportive.

5. Within this atmosphere of consistency and predictability the young child also benefits from experiences of variety and contrast. Such experiences sharpen perception and awareness, creating those mild psychological tensions that call for an adaptive response. When the tension is not so great as to overwhelm and disorganize the child, a novel experience or stimulus can enhance development in a number of ways.

6. The child needs toys and other playthings. While a responsive human partner is crucial to the child's development, he also needs toys that can be used independently and with others. In addition to their usefulness for intellectual growth, toys serve an important function in the child's emotional life. One of their advantages is their emotional neutrality; a child can use them in many ways to work out

feelings and develop ideas without evoking an emotional response from the toy.

7. The child needs limits, prohibitions, and expectations for conformity from the adults. These are beneficial when provided in an atmosphere of continuity and affectionate attention. Harshness, coldness, and severe punishment have no place in rearing a healthy young child, but it is also believed that development cannot proceed in a favorable way for a child whose parents are markedly overindulgent, excessively permissive, or extremely inconsistent in what they require of him. Setting reasonable limits and imposing reasonable requirements are as much a part of loving a child and supporting his development as are feeding, cuddling, and speaking to him.

These, then, are some of the general characteristics of a supportive environment. When there are disturbances in the child's development, however, a high degree of individualization of care, that is, a specific prescription, can be of great importance in alleviating problems. The therapeutic task requires that the person providing care know the child patient well and be able to modify, extend, or emphasize certain types of care or certain specific experiences for the child.

In discussing the application of research on parent-child relationships, I shall first present in condensed form some of the work of psychoanalytic clinicians and investigators. Psychoanalytic developmental psychology assigns central importance in the child's personality development to his relationships with other persons; the study of human object relations has been a dominant concern of analysis from the beginning. Freud (1926) outlined two stages in the child's development of human relationships: the need for the gratifying, comfort-giving, that is, the anaclitic object, and the later need for the permanent object. Many psychoanalytic clinicians and investigators, among them Hartmann, Kris, and Loewenstein (1946), Kris (1951), A. Freud (1965), Fraiberg (1969), Mahler, Pine, and Bergman (1975), Spitz (1965), have contributed to the literature on these two overlapping phases and have identified subphases within them.

The prolonged dependency of the human infant, his need for care and protection not only for survival but for the experiences essential to development and learning, intensify the importance of the child's nurturers and enormously enhance their significance for his psychological development. The mother's relationship to her infant is both biological and social. The infant's social and emotional needs are met in close association with the mother's response to his bodily needs. In infancy and early childhood the influences of the society and culture are mediated primarily through the nurturing adults and are gradually augmented through the child's relationships with significant others. The child begins to form his first attachment to the person who is able to understand and satisfy his basic needs. The importance of continuity and consistency of the principal caregiver to optimize development is generally agreed upon in psychoanalysis. The mother, who is the provider of many experiences of comfort, satisfaction, and pleasure for the child, is also the source of prohibitions, discomfort, and frustrating experiences in the normal course of their daily lives together. All of these experiences are important for the child's development. Anna Freud (1965), in summarizing much that has been learned from clinical investigation, has emphasized that interference with the mother-infant tie by any cause or by failure of the mother to play her part as a reliable, need-fulfilling, and comfort-giving person may interfere with subsequent development in a variety of ways.

The benevolence, reliability, and continuity of the nurturing person are important not only because the infant's physical and psychosocial needs are best met through such nurturing, but also because such care facilitates development in general. To mention only a few examples: such mental functions as discrimination between things and persons in the environment, the psychological investment in sensorimotor experiences, and the distinction between inner and outer stimuli depend in important ways on the quality of object relationships. Such ego functions as motility, perception, speech, and intelligence may be enhanced or impeded according to the adequacy of the young child's object relations; attitudes toward reality are deeply influenced by object relations; and trouble in object relations often interferes with another important function of the ego, the formation of stable defenses. Object relations are a crucial co-determinant of instinctual drive development, its organization and behavioral expression. On the other hand, all of these ego and instinctual factors participate in the development of the object relationship. For example, the infant's and young child's ability first to recognize the mother and others and later to "read" nonverbal cues or understand speech contains significant cognitive elements. Similarly, it is believed that the infant's drive endowment and differentiation, among other congenital characteristics, in part determine his individual needs and developmental tendencies including the character of his object relations. Psychoanalytic developmental psychology thus employs a complex theory and asks that one avoid the pitfalls of oversimplification of the content of the human mind, even that of the very young child.

The child's relationships especially with his parents also influence his relations to inanimate objects during the early years of life. Based on some of her studies of severely deprived infants in foundling homes, Katherine Wolf (1948) emphasized that the infant's coming to believe in inanimate objects (a world of things), that is, to have a memory of their consistency and constancy, depends upon the consistency and constancy of the human object. Later investigations, including the study of infants in institutions that Rose Lipton and I published (1962), provided data that supported Wolf's point of view. Samuel Ritvo and I discussed (1961) some of the disturbances in the use of toys seen in these institutional infants. The interpersonal relationship between infant and parent is an important source of interest in toys, and the parents' pleasure in the baby's activity with the toy further promotes his own pleasure in it. Those who work with or know infants and young children are familiar with how an adult's enthusiasm for a toy or an activity makes it attractive to the child. Such knowledge is used frequently in stimulating the interest of a child who is apathetic or indifferent, or whom one wants to help with learning or with play.

In addition, the opportunity for play with toys in an atmosphere in which there is not perpetual competition from the adult has proved to be another important factor. An atmosphere of constant, high emotional charge does not, in our experience, promote the adaptive use of toys and learning through play. The influence of the child's relationship with mother and later with other trustworthy persons on playful activity, both social play and play with toys, has significant application to clinical work. Early childhood specialists know, of course, that a young child who cannot play in a manner appropriate to his age and culture is a child who is in psychological difficulty. In diagnostic work we rely heavily on what we can learn about the child's mental life—his intellectual ability, conflicts, fantasies, interests, ideas and personal style—by observing the child's play, and when we set about to help him, one of our most reliable methods is to play with him.

Recent studies of newborn infants or newborns and their parents have either extended or made more explicit some of the empirical knowledge clinicians have used. For example, studies by Louis Sander (1962, 1970) with newborns and their mothers demonstrated the influence of the members of the dyad on one another's behavior. Among the fascinating aspects of Sander's work are observations of the influence of variations in maternal caretaking behavior on the biological rhythms of the child which traditionally are presumed to be entirely innately determined. Sander's emphasis on the conceptual framework that includes the intrinsic subsystems of the infant, the infant as a whole—that is, his integrative capacities or state and the extrinsic caretaking environment—is important. Similarly, some of the work of Brazelton and his colleagues (1974) having to do with mother-infant (and father-infant) interaction in the early days of life demonstrates the complexity of that interaction even then. Daniel Stern (1973) has documented some of the subtleties of how mother and infant make and avoid eye contact and influence each other with exchanges of such brief duration that they might pass unnoticed on ordinary observation. Leiderman and Seashore (1975), in their studies of healthy premature babies and their mothers, found significant differences in the mother-child relationship in those who were separated early compared with those in which mothers had early contact as caregivers. This has been an interesting and valuable confirmation of what has been observed more informally for some time, that is, it can indeed make an important difference in how the mother-infant relationship develops when the mother begins to take care of her infant as soon as possible. The work of Klaus and Kennell (1976) in a hospital setting emphasizes the importance to the mother-child relationship of the active support of physicians, nurses, and other hospital personnel in facilitating the attachment, and these authors make a strong plea for more support for mothers in the early days of their infants' lives.

Some of the studies are fine examples of aspects of what Erikson (1950) referred to as mutuality (or the mutual adaptation) of a mother and her infant. Some of them reexamine, illustrate, or make more explicit aspects of the kind of care of infants and parents that was provided in the pioneering demonstration and research project of Edith Jackson, Ethelyn Klatskin, and their colleagues in the rooming-in project at Yale in the 1950s (Klatskin and Jackson, 1955). The project was based on the assumption that a benevolent and supportive environment provided by skilled clinicians could make a difference in how parents understood and nurtured their young children and in their development as parents.

The many studies on separation as well as those on loss of parents have been of great influence in determining the organization and performance of therapeutic efforts with infants and young children (Freud and Burlingham, 1944; Spitz, 1946, 1950; Spitz and Wolf, 1946; Bowlby, 1951, 1973; Benjamin, 1963; Yarrow, 1964; Mahler, 1966; Wallerstein and Kelly, 1975). Studies of infants without families, loss of one parent through death or divorce, studies of children in multiple placements are examples of these well-known studies. There is little argument about whether such separation or loss has an impact on the infant's psychological development. The questions and disagreements concern the extent of the influence of these events, the specific aspects of the child's mental and emotional life that are affected, and the effect of such experiences on subsequent development.

Another area of research that has proved to have important clinical applications is the study of anxiety in infancy and early childhood. The typical phases of developmental anxiety in the child described by Freud in 1926 and elaborated by many others are closely linked with and reflect the nature of the child's relationships with emotionally important adults. During the early years, the fear of loss of the person to whom the child is attached as the primary nurturer can be seen from the last quarter of the first year onward and is followed by the fear of loss of that person's love and approval. Indeed the young child's wish, at least a large part of the time, to please and be approved of by his parents is the strongest single force in the socialization process which enables him to become a reasonably healthy, participating member of his family, his peer group, and the larger society. Among the more meticulous studies of developmental anxiety were those of Spitz (1950), and later of Benjamin (1961, 1963) based upon observations of infants and interpreted primarily in the framework of psychoanalysis. Benjamin in particular pointed out some of the individual variations among infants and young children, and he put forth several hypotheses about some of the determinants of exaggerated manifestations of such anxiety. We use some of these ideas when we understand and try to alleviate anxieties that occur when children are hospitalized or separated from their parents for other reasons.

Other studies important in developing the conceptual framework for organizing a therapeutic environment for disturbed young children are those of variations in inborn tendencies of infants and their influence on development. Perhaps the clearest statements of the possible implications of these differences have come from the work of Sybille Escalona and are set out in her book, *The Roots of Individuality* (1968). The influence of the child's congenital characteristics on parental reactions to him, some of the ways in which mother and infant shape each other's behavior, the dynamic nature of the interactional process and its multiple determinants are carefully examined in Escalona's studies.

Another relevant area of study has been the effect of sensory defects on the development of the relationship between parent and child and the impact of that relationship on various dimensions of the child's development. One of the most valuable examples is the work of

Selma Fraiberg and her colleagues (1969, 1971) in a longitudinal study of the development of blind children. The impact of the child's blindness on parental attitudes and behavior with the child is one aspect of the problem. Both the parents' need for assistance and their response have been documented. The importance of providing not only emotional satisfaction and social experiences but experiences with toys and other inanimate objects and, as Fraiberg puts it, to "educate the hands" of the blind child, has also been demonstrated. As the children grew older, the Fraiberg group's data showed that in well-nurtured blind children the bonding or emotional attachment to the mother could develop quite appropriately, and yet, because of the blindness, the child's ability to develop the concept of object permanence in Piaget's sense was interfered with. If the mother was not within reach or sound, the infant and toddler could experience this as a loss of the mother in a way that engendered panic states in many of them. Fraiberg's examination of Psychoanalytic theory of object relationships and Piaget's theory of the development of object permanence as an aspect of sensorimotor intelligence illustrate the complementarity and usefulness of the two theories in the clinical approach to a specific problem.

As one example of how knowledge from a number of sources might influence clinical practice one could cite what we have learned about language development. Theories and assertions about the way language development occurs in the child have varied all the way from the idea that it is uninfluenced by the environment to the notion that it is almost completely determined by the child's environment. Many studies by clinicians and other child development specialists have examined various aspects of language development, and one can find persuasive data both for the importance of intrinsic equipmental and maturational factors and for the child's experience, particularly with other persons (Brodbeck and Irwin, 1946; Lewis, 1959; Provence and Lipton, 1962; Lenneberg, 1967; Nelson, 1973; de Hirsch, 1975). One of the more exciting additions in recent years came not from child-development research but from Noam Chomsky (Lyons, 1970) who introduced into our conceptual framework of language development the theory that speaking includes an internal process of transformation and generativity. His ideas have profoundly influenced both linguistics and the aspect of psychology that is concerned with children's language. Eric Lenneberg (1967) extended some of these ideas, discussing the importance of these tranformational and generative processes in the child's learning to speak and to understand the language of others. Lenneberg emphasized the importance of species-specific biological attributes in the development of speech, which do not negate the importance of the speaking environment of the child nor the vital role of the child's object relationships in his verbal communication.

In regard to cognitive development, also, these transformational and generative characteristics have been emphasized by Peter Wolff (1969), who wrote, ". . . children have at their disposal unlearned, or at least unteachable, acquisition devices for creating order out of random events and for transforming ordered experience into generative principles (cognitive structures)" (p. 18).

In discussing very briefly a few things about the support for parents in their development as parents, I simply want to be sure to include the fact that parenthood, too, is a developmental process. In clinical work, because we are trying to understand what has gone wrong in the developmental process or why the child has a psychiatric disturbance or some developmental delay, we focus a good deal of attention and energy on trying to understand what, in the parents' own lives and in the way they behave with the child, might be the most important determinant of the picture brought to us. I have no criticism of that; indeed, it is a necessary part of diagnosis and of devising an effective therapeutic plan. Sometimes, however, we do not pay enough attention to the strengths that parents bring; our evaluations should contain more of that kind of assessment and thinking. In addition, we need to be more steady and creative in helping parents to understand their child and to support their development as parents. While we must be mindful of their needs as adults outside of their role as parents, the mental health field in general has deemphasized its earlier gift for counseling of parents through sharing knowledge of their children and helping parents to find solutions.

Among the necessary conditions for clinical work with the individual child is a careful evaluation of the child and his situation: the collection of diagnostic data through clinical interviewing of parents on more than one occasion, a comprehensive developmental assessment of the child, and the observation of parents and child together. The synthesis of data from all sources and the formulation of the diagnosic statement are necessary preconditions to the most specific, individualized approach to the child. From such an evaluation one should be able to develop a specific profile of the child's functioning —his developmental strengths as well as the deficits—and to create a therapeutic plan for him. This can be done even when one does not entirely understand the genesis of the problem. Then one must watch the child, modifying the plan in response to changing needs.

In our case load, problems originating in disturbances in parent-child relationships are very common and take many forms: children who do not grow normally, children who have vomiting or diarrhea or other body symptoms, children whose speech is impaired, children whose behavior gets them in trouble with their parents or other adults, children who are recognizably depressed or unusually anxious, children who are lacking in the expected capacities for self-regulation and impulse control, children who cannot cope with the normal stresses of everyday life; children whose relationships to others are characterized by lack of discrimination or mistrust or confusion, children whose intellectual development is delayed or very uneven, children whose control over their own bodies is impaired in some way. These are among the frequently found indicators of psychological disturbances, but they must be distinguished from other conditions which cause the same symptoms.

The clinical work necessarily involves work with the parents, with parent substitutes, with other caregivers and teachers. Direct work with a young child, while not unknown, has not been done as much as I personally would like to see. Even in situations in which it is clear that help for the infant or young child primarily depends on the ability to help the parents, there is much to be said for clinician's either working regularly with the child or having enough direct knowledge of the child to individualize the recommendations.

The settings in which the clinical work is done vary. One thinks first of developmental and mental health clinics for the very young, of hospital wards, and increasingly of daycare centers and nursery schools. However, much of the work can also be effectively done in the patient's own home. The choice of setting should be related to the specific situation of the child and his family. My plea is for flexibility in that regard.

A condensed version of an extensive evaluation followed by a treatment plan is given to illustrate some of the points made in the previous pages.

> Charles was 18 months old when he and his mother, Mrs. B., were referred to us by his pediatrician because of an intractable sleep problem. He was the third child and first boy to be born to his parents. Named after his father who abandoned the family when Charles was three months old, Charles was described by his mother as an irritable infant who demanded much attention from her. Although she enjoyed him and felt close to him in many respects, we gradually learned that she identified him in part with the charming and cruel husband who had abandoned her. She was able to tell us that she often felt controlled by the baby and feared he would grow up to be just like his father. In a series of interviews that paralleled the evaluation of the child, we learned that, except for the problem with Charles, she and her daughters were coping reasonably well. They had considerable psychological support from Mrs. B.'s parents and siblings. Our evaluation of her revealed her to be a person who had no severe psychopathology, was eager for help and ready to work on her relationship with Charles.
>
> The evaluation of Charles revealed that, besides his sleep problem, his development was in considerable disharmony. He was motorically active and reasonably competent in gross motor skills. Language was moderately delayed; he was unable to play in a manner expected at his age. While he was obviously strongly attached to his mother and sisters, he interacted with them largely in imperious and demanding ways or cried bitterly when he wanted something. His frustration tolerance was very low. He often broke his toys. No attempt had been made to toilet-train him. The sleep problem had, his mother said, been going on "all his life."
>
> Our proposal to the mother was that she and Charles work

with us for a time. Charles was seen twice a week by one of our nursery school teachers who was able to be both empathic and firm. She was a facilitator of play and a playmate for him, helping him to become interested in a variety of play materials. During these sessions she also talked with him a great deal about what he was doing and feeling. She limited his behavior when he endangered himself and helped him channel his aggressive impulses. As his interests widened and competence increased, he was much less imperious, both with his teacher and at home, and his excitement and tantrums diminished. He and his mother came to share many more pleasurable times, he expressed a greater variety of feelings, he was able to talk to her and to others much more effectively, which gave him great satisfaction.

Mrs. B. saw her social worker once a week and attended Charles' session with his teacher once a week.

The exchange of information and close coordination of the work of the social worker and teacher with Mrs. B. and Charles made for an effective intervention. Mrs. B. was able to understand how her identification of Charles with her husband had influenced her care, and to modify it. The work with Charles made it easier for mother and child to enjoy each other more and enhanced the child's general development. After a four-month treatment, we considered that they were in no further need of help. Mrs. B. knows that the clinic is available should she wish to consult us in the future.

In working therapeutically with young children and their parents, everyone uses some theoretical approach, has some conceptual framework that provides guidelines to action, whether or not it is spelled out.

For the very young child, there is no doubt that the therapeutic environment leans heavily on the proposition that a benevolent, reasonably mature and caring adult is the necessary provider and mediator of this environment. In addition, there is a steadily growing body of knowledge about childhood disorders, about variability in children, about methods of influencing specific problems, and about working with parents which is useful and often effective.

REFERENCES

BENJAMIN, J. 1961. Some developmental observations relating to the theory of anxiety. *J. Am. Psychoanal. Assoc.*, 9:652-668.

BENJAMIN, J. 1963. Further comments on some developmental aspects of anxiety. In H. S. Gaskill (ed.), *Counterpoint: Libidinal Object and Subject*, pp. 121-153. New York: International Universities Press.

BOWLBY, J. 1951. *Maternal Care and Mental Health*. Geneva: World Health Organization Monograph No. 2.

BOWLBY, J. 1973. *Attachment and Loss*, vol. 2. New York: Basic Books.

BRAZELTON, T. B., KOSLOWSKI, B., and MAIN, M. 1974. The origins of reciprocity: The early mother-infant interaction. In M. Lewis and L. Rosenblum (eds.), *The Origins of Behavior*, vol. 1, pp. 49-76. New York: Wiley.

BRODBECK, A. J., and IRWIN, O. C. 1946. The speech behavior of infants without families. *Child Devel.*, 17:145-156.

DE HIRSCH, K. 1975. Language deficits in children with development lags. *Psychoanal. Study Child*, 30:95-126.

ERIKSON, E. 1950. *Childhood and Society*. New York: Norton.

ESCALONA, S. 1968. *The Roots of Individuality*. Chicago: Aldine.

FRAIBERG, S. 1969. Libidinal object constancy and mental representation. *Psychoanal. Study Child*, 19:133-169.

FRAIBERG, S. 1971. Separation crisis in two blind children. *Psychoanal. Study Child*, 26:355-371.

FREUD, A. 1965. *Normality and Pathology in Childhood: Assessments of Development*, pp. 64-66. New York: International Universities Press.

FREUD, A., and BURLINGHAM, D. 1944. *Infants Without Families*. New York: International Universities Press.

FREUD, S. 1926. Inhibitions, symptoms and anxiety. *Standard Ed.*, 20:77-175.

HARTMANN, H., KRIS, E., and LOEWENSTEIN, R. M. 1946. Comments on the formation of psychic structure. *Psychoanal. Study Child*, 2:11-38.

KLATSKIN, E. H., and JACKSON, E. B. 1955. Methodology of the Yale rooming-in project on parent-child relationship. *Am J. Orthopsychiatry*, 25:81-104.

KLAUS, M. H., and KENNELL, J. H. 1976. *Maternal-Infant Bonding*. St. Louis: Mosby.

KRIS, E. 1951. Opening remarks on psychoanalytic child psychology. *Psychoanal. Study Child*, 6:9-17.

LEIDERMAN, P. H., and SEASHORE, M. J. 1975. Mother-infant neonatal separation: Some delayed consequences. In Ciba Foundation Symposium 33, *Parent-Infant Interaction*, pp. 213-239. Amsterdam: ASP.

LENNEBERG, E. 1967. The biological fundations of language. *Hospital Practice*, 2:59-67.

LEWIS, M. M. 1959. *How Children Learn to Speak*. New York: Basic Books.

LYONS, J. 1970. *Noam Chomsky*. New York: Viking Press.

MAHLER, M. 1966. Notes on the development of basic moods: The depressive affect. In R. M. Loewenstein, K. R. Eissler, et al. (eds.), *Psychoanalysis: A General Psychology*, pp. 152-168. New York: International Universities Press.

MAHLER, M., PINE, F., and BERGMAN, A. (eds.). 1975. *The Psychological Birth of the Human Infant*. New York: Basic Books.

NELSON, K. 1973. *Structure and Strategy in Learning to Talk*. Monograph Serial No. 149. Chicago: University of Chicago Press.

PROVENCE, S. 1967. *A Guide to the Care of Infants in Groups*. New York: Child Welfare League.

PROVENCE, S. 1968. The first year of life: The infant. In L. Dittman (ed.), *Early Child Care*, pp. 27-39. New York: Atherton.

PROVENCE, S. 1972. Psychoanalysis and the treatment of psychological disorders of infancy. In B. Wolman (ed.), *Handbook of Child Psychoanalysis*, pp. 191-220. New York: Van Nostrand Reinhold.

PROVENCE, S., and LIPTON, R. 1962. *Infants in Institutions*. New York: International Universities Press.

PROVENCE, S., and RITVO, S. 1961. Effects of deprivation on institutionalized infants. *Psychoanal. Study Child*, 16:189-205.

SANDER, L. 1962. Issues in early mother-child interaction. *J. Am. Acad. Child Psychiatry*, 1:141-166.

SANDER, L. 1970. Early mother-infant interaction and 24-hour patterns of activity and sleep. *J. Am. Acad. Child Psychiatry*, 9:103-123.

SPITZ, R. 1946. Hospitalism: A follow-up report. *Psychoanal. Study Child*, 2:113-117.

SPITZ, R. 1950. Anxiety in infancy: A study of its manifestations in the first year of life. *Int. J. Psychoanal.*, 31:138-143.

SPITZ, R. 1965. *The First Year of Life*. New York: International Universities Press.

SPITZ, R., and WOLF, K. M. 1946. Anaclitic depression: An inquiry into the genesis of psychiatric conditions in early childhood. *Psychoanal. Study Child*, 2:313-342.

STERN, D. N. 1973. Mother and infant at play: The dyadic interaction involving facial, vocal and gaze behaviors. In M. Lewis and L. Rosenblum (eds.), *The Origins of Behavior*, vol. 1, pp. 187-213. New York: Wiley.

WALLERSTEIN, J. S., and KELLY, J. B. 1975. The effects of parental divorce. *J. Am. Acad. Child Psychiatry*, 14:600-616.

WOLF, K. M. 1948. Unpublished seminar notes.

WOLFF, P. 1969. What we must and must not teach our young children from what we know about early cognitive development. In P. H. Wolff and R. McKeith (eds.), *Planning for Better Learning*, p. 18. London: Heinemann.

YARROW, L. 1964. Separation from parents during early childhood. In M. L. Hoffman and L. W. Hoffman (eds.), *Review of Child Development Research*, pp. 89-136. New York: Russell Sage Foundation.

13

Development of Childhood Deviance: A Study of 223 Urban Black Men from Birth to 18

LEE N. ROBINS, Ph.D.

and

ERIC WISH, Ph.D.

Behaviors in childhood that can be labeled as deviant, antisocial, or conduct problems are of great interest both intrinsically, because of the difficulties they cause parents, teachers, peers, and the community, and as predictors of many aspects of adult life. Many studies, including our own (Robins, 1966), have shown that antisocial children have greatly increased risks of a large number of undesirable adult outcomes including incarceration, unemployment, marital instability, impoverished interpersonal relationships, addiction to alcohol and illicit drugs, psychiatric care, and early death. It is also true, however, that much deviant behavior of childhood is occasional and transient. We know that the more varied and frequent the deviance of childhood, the greater the risk of its predicting later maladjustment, but we know very little so far about how childhood deviance *becomes* varied and frequent. While there are well-substantiated correlations between the *occurrence* of some types of deviance and background factors such as parental deviance, dis-

This paper was supported by U.S.P.H.S. Grants MH 18864, DA 4RG 008, DA 00259, and Research Scientist Award DA 00013.

turbed homes, delinquent siblings, and poverty, these factors alone and in combination do not seem to explain satisfactorily how far a child will go in exploring varieties of possible deviance. Nor does the social-control system by which deviance is punished appear a satisfactory explanation for its termination.

What should we make of the fact that some children exhibit a great variety of deviant behaviors? It could have several meanings. First, we could be misled. Committing deviant acts might be a purely random process, in which we identify children in the tail of a chance distribution as distinct only when they cross a "badness" threshold that we impose on the facts as observers.

Second, it could mean that some children are intrinsically more at risk of deviance than others, whether as a result of genetic or environmental influences or both. This predisposition to deviance might be one of three types—a general predisposition to do whatever is socially disapproved, no matter what it is (i.e., the children might be "bad apples"); a susceptibility to one special form of deviance, such as truancy, which when added to other types of deviance that occur by chance makes us perceive the children as indulging in an unusual variety of disapproved behaviors; or a tendency to act precociously, in which case the children are called deviant because they do while still children what most people wait to do until adulthood.

Third, deviance may have its own developmental process, which once started leads from one type of deviance to another, unless social controls effectively interrupt it. That developmental process may be a quantitative one, in which the likelihood of committing an untried deviant act depends principally on the number of other types of deviance already tried, or a qualitative one, where certain specific acts are necessary or nearly necessary stepping stones to others.

We can be reasonably sure that childhood deviance is not a purely random process because we can predict fairly accurately which young children will be deviant. We do this in two ways—one consistent with the "predisposition" hypothesis, the other with the "developmental" hypothesis. When we predict that children of inadequate parents and from impoverished neighborhoods will be deviant, we are assuming that they have a genetically or environmentally produced predisposition. When we predict that children who disobey the teacher in first grade will be delinquents, we are inferring that there is a natural progression from one type of deviance to another —that is, a developmental process. Of course, we may be incorrect in this inference of progression, because it may simply be that the same genetic and environmental factors predict both types of deviance.

The purpose of this paper is to examine to what extent there is evidence for a developmental process in childhood deviance. Describing that process, if it exists, has both theoretical and practical importance. On the theoretical level, it should assist in integrating the study of deviant behavior into the field of child development, which has long concentrated almost entirely on *positive* achievements: physical growth, neurological maturation, and the acquisition of intellectual skills. On the practical level, it could suggest both the degree of urgency and the best timing of intervention to prevent progression from less serious to more serious forms of deviant behavior.

To discern whether there is evidence for a developmental process of deviance and, if so, whether it is both a quantitative process, in which committing any one deviant behavior makes all others more likely, and a qualitative one, in which committing certain specific behaviors makes committing another specific behavior more likely, we will use the age-dated initiations of 13 deviant behaviors during the childhoods of 223 young black men to study the patterns and sequencing of deviance.

We will begin by defining the behaviors selected as deviant and showing their frequency and the range of ages at which they first occurred. We will then demonstrate what we already strongly suspect —that the number of deviant behaviors per child is not the product of a purely random process.

Next we will consider what kinds of correlations should be expected among acts beginning at various ages and affecting varying proportions of a population if there is a developmental process, and if it is (a) quantitative or (b) qualitative. If the findings are consistent with a developmental pattern, we will next try to establish *which* acts lead to which other acts. To do this, we will need to take into account their order of appearance, while controlling for variation in the periods at risk and variation in the number and types of other behaviors that may render apparent causal relationships spurious. Once we have established what seem to be causal connections between behaviors, we will evaluate their practical importance for those interested in prediction or intervention.

In the present paper we will not try to compare the importance of a developmental process with the importance of either predispositions to deviance (whether inborn or environmentally created) or of social controls in determining the choice of deviant acts or the likelihood of transitions from one form of deviance to another. Obviously predisposition and social controls are extremely important. But they are also the focus of most prior research on deviance, our own along with that of others. It is rather on the long-neglected topic of deviance as a developmental process in its own right that we will focus, leaving a broader integration for the future.

METHODS

In our earlier study (Robins, 1966), in which we first investigated which behavior problems of childhood predicted adult deviance, we did not have the data necessary to study a developmental process because the child guidance clinic records which provided the childhood histories did not systematically date the onsets of these behaviors. Without date of onset, one cannot study the transitions from one behavior to the next. Further, the subjects in that study for whom we had detailed childhood information* had all been referred to a clinic, and were therefore by definition deviant. This meant that we could not investigate early-childhood deviance that terminates before it is serious enough to call for referral to court or clinic.

---

* The study also includes a small normal control group for whom we had school records as well as interviews, but the controls had been selected for an absence of serious school problems and in addition lacked the detailed social and behavioral histories available in the clinic records. Thus, they were not a sample in which we could study the development of childhood deviance.

(We did, however, find many subjects whose childhood deviance did not carry over into adulthood.) Finally, the clinic histories were taken at the point of first clinic contact, usually age 13 or 14, and thus were incomplete for late adolescent behaviors.

The present paper is part of a study of normal black men which was designed to replicate some aspects of the first study and to remedy some of its defects. Since this study is based on a general population sample rather than a clinic sample, it provides both deviant and nondeviant children. Further, in interview as adults, each subject was asked about the age of initiation of each of the childhood behaviors about which we inquired, which makes it possible to study their sequence of onsets. The current study, however, also has its limitations. The sample is small (N=223) and homogeneous, in that it consists entirely of urban-born-and-reared black American males born in the early 1930s in St. Louis. Thus there are problems in generalizing from this sample to other populations. The study investigates only 13 deviant behaviors out of the many one could imagine investigating. Information about the age of onset of some of these behaviors comes from school and police records, which were made contemporaneously with the commission of the behaviors and so must be correct. For the other behaviors, age at onset was obtained by retrospection at about age 33. Obviously these men did not always correctly recall the age of first occurrence of each of these behaviors. However, ages reported seem to have some validity, since we found age of reported first alcohol and first drug use to be powerful predictors of both self-reported and record indicators of degree of adult drug and alcohol involvement (Robins and Murphy, 1967; Robins et al., 1968).

It is possible, of course, that men may have omitted telling us about some of their childhood deviance entirely. However, the checking of police records has given evidence that the validity of at least some of their statements about past deviance is remarkably high. For instance, every man who had a police or Federal Bureau of Narcotics record indicating heroin abuse reported heroin use in interview. Thus we have reason to believe that intentional denial of childhood deviance was not an important problem.

We are also optimistic about the generalizability of our findings despite the small homogeneous sample, since we have already shown that the childhood predictors of adult psychiatric status in this sample are very similar to those discovered in our previous study of whites of an older generation (Robins et al., 1971).

Selection of the Sample

The criteria for eligibility for the study were being male, born in St. Louis between 1930 and 1934, attending for six years or more a St. Louis public elementary school serving the black community, having an intelligence quotient (IQ) score of at least 85 while in elementary school, and guardian's name and occupation appearing on the school record. The total population of eligible boys was 930; 240 of these were initially selected for follow-up. The sample was designed to provide 30 men in each of the eight categories created by taking all combinations of three dichotomized school-record variables: father's presence or absence, guardian's occupation at the lowest level versus a higher level, moderate or severe school problems versus mild problems or none. The distributions of IQ scores, year of birth, and number of addresses at which the boys were known to have lived during elementary school were matched across all eight groups. The level of breadwinner's occupation and the distribution of the nature and seriousness of elementary-school problems were matched across the four groups composing each half of a dichotomy in order to avoid, for example, children from intact homes being predominantly grade repeaters, while children from broken homes were predominantly truants. Additional matching was done within the halves of the father-present-or-absent dichotomy for the father's continued absence or presence when the boy reached high school.

Men who had not lived in the St. Louis area at all during the last six years were discarded from the sample and replaced by the best matching of the remaining pool of eligible cases. A statement by a relative or by the man himself, or a death certificate before 1959, was required as evidence of a man's not meeting the residence criterion. Because of nonresidence or death, 87 men were eliminated.

In the category "father absent, high occupation and no school problems" all eligible cases were exhausted, leaving only 25 instead of the desired 30 cases in this category. The final sample, then, consists of 235 men whose elementary-school records showed half with school problems, half without; half with father in the home, half without; half with guardians who were unemployed, domestic servants or laborers, and half with guardians in better jobs; all with IQs of 85 or higher and all born in St. Louis between 1930 and 1934.

The sample selection procedures were relevant to the general purposes of the study—to test hypotheses about the independent effects of social class, antisocial fathers, and own early deviance on adult adjustment—but are not relevant to the issues which the present paper addresses.

Because the sample was selected in this special way, it was weighted properly to make it representative of the population from which it was selected—black males born in St. Louis between 1930-1934 who attended public school for at least six years and who had an IQ of 85 or higher. Because we had collected school records of all eligible cases, and divided them into the eight selection groups obtained by taking all combinations of three dichotomies—high and low occupation, school problems or none, father present or absent, it was easy to calculate the weights that would make the sample representative of the eligible population. It should be remembered, however, that the eligible population itself is a special one.

In 1965 and 1966 interviews were obtained for 223 of these young men, 221 with them personally and two with relatives of men who had died within the six years prior to interview. The current paper deals with information only about those for whom interviews were obtained, omitting the 12 (5 percent) who are unlocated or refused an interview. Since all these young men grew up in the same urban community, the school and police records provide a quite complete set of data from which to assess their school behavior and juvenile arrest histories.

The Deviant Acts

The deviant behavior to be discussed concerns the commission of 13 types of acts. The behaviors to be considered are: (1) elementary school academic problems (FAIL), defined as elementary school records showing at least three quarters held back, and at least one of these in grade three or later—or placement in special class or school for the educationally handicapped; (2) behavior problems in elementary school (ABSENCE) as indicated by school records showing more than 20 percent of school days missed in at least five quarters, at least one of these in grade three or later, or notations of truancy or expulsion or transfer to a reformatory; (3) leaving school before graduation from high school (DROPOUT), as indicated on school records by permanent withdrawal before high school graduation or temporary withdrawal for a semester or more; (4) juvenile offense (ARREST), as indicated by a police record of an offense prior to age 18 or juvenile court record resulting from the child's own misbehavior (records resulting from parental neglect, adoption, or temporary placement are not included); (5) precocious use of alcohol (DRINK) defined as interview reports of taking a first drink of alcohol before the age of 15; (6) precocious sexual experience (SEX) as indicated by interview report of first intercourse before the age of 15; (7) use of marijuana before age 18 (MARJ); (8) use of barbiturates before age 18 (BARB); (9) use of amphetamines before age 18 (AMPH); (10) use of opiates before age 18 (OPIATE); (11) leaving the parental home to live on his own before age 18 (LEFT HOME); (12) marriage before age 18 (MARRIAGE); and (13) developing alcohol problems such as "the shakes" or family complaints before age 18 (ALC PROB). As noted above, the first four of these variables come from records, the remainder from retrospective report at time of interview.

It will be noted that sex and drinking were counted only if they occurred before age 15. This age was chosen because after 15 both behaviors were so common that it was hard to believe that they could have been considered deviant in the local subculture. Failure and absence also have a cut-off age below 15 because children were no longer in elementary school after that time.

School problems present a unique difficulty in assigning a time of initiation. Children can be occasionally absent or temporarily behind their classmates in achievement without being considered by the school as having a problem. They are considered to have school problems only when they have *recurrent* difficulties. Yet when a sequence of behaviors is required to meet the criterion for a problem, when does the problem "begin"—when the child takes the first step that eventuates in his meeting the criterion or when he takes the final step that puts him over the criterion threshold? We decided to accept the former definition, assessing academic and behavior problems on the basis of the whole elementary school record, and for those who qualified as having had problems at some time during elementary school, counting the earliest age at which that problem behavior appeared. Thus, the child who was eventually put in an ungraded room is counted as deviant the first time he is held back, and the child who becomes chronically truant is called deviant as of the age he first misses 20 percent of school days in one school quarter. It may seem odd to consider school failure as a form of deviance. It should be remembered, however, that all members of the sample had shown IQ scores of at least 85, a level more than adequate for progressing normally through elementary school.

For behaviors other than sex, drinking, absence, and failure, the upper limit was the end of the childhood period, age 18.

RESULTS

Frequency and Age of Initiation for 13 Behaviors

The 13 behaviors varied considerably in frequency, age of first initiation, and whether they occurred predominantly early or late in the age span at risk. Table 1 shows that the number of children committing these behaviors varied in frequency from 56 percent who had sexual experience before 15 to only 3 percent who used opiates before 18. (As we showed in a previous paper [Robins and Murphy, 1967], 12 percent of these men eventually did use heroin, but the median age of beginning use was 19 years, which is past our cut-off for "childhood.")

The beginning ages of elementary school failure and absence were determined by age of school entry at six, and marriage, which

TABLE 1

Deviant Behaviors in Childhood
(223 Young Black Men)

	Proportion Doing This (%)	Age Range of Initiations	Median Age at Initiation
SEX	56	4-14	13.1
ABSENCE	43	6-14	7.3
DROPOUT	39	6-17	16.2
ARREST	38	5-17	15.2
FAIL	34	6-13	7.7
DRINK	34	2-14	13.1
LEFT HOME	26	8-17	17.2
MARIJUANA	20	8-17	15-7
MARRIAGE	6	14-17	17.5
BARBS	6	11-17	16.5
ALC PROB	5	14-17	16.7
AMPHS	4	13-17	15.8
OPIATES	3	12-17	17.1

waited on puberty, did not occur before 14. Alcohol problems had to wait on some drinking experience. Otherwise, there were no absolute lower limits (as the not infrequent prepubertal sex experience shows). Sex, drinking, and arrests occurred in rare children even before school age, and first marijuana use and leaving home also occasionally occurred very early. Other drug-use and alcohol problems occurred only in adolescence.

Elementary school problems were distinct from other behaviors in that they began early or not at all. Before their eighth birthday, more than half the children who would ever be seriously held back or truant had already been so. For all other behaviors, frequencies were low at first and gradually accelerated. If we count as the period at risk the ages from when the first child committed a behavior to the cut-off dates at 15 and 18, we find that, except for elementary

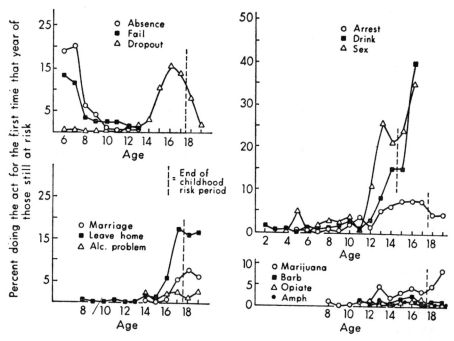

FIGURE 1. Percentage of those at risk of beginning a new form of deviance who did so each year.

school problems, the majority of first occurrences of all other behaviors were in the last three years of the period at risk. The behaviors that occurred last of all were opiate use, leaving home, and marrying.

The accumulation of initiations at the end of their risk periods suggested that these behaviors were not restricted to childhood, and that those not showing them before 18 might well do so soon after. To see whether this was so, we extended our look at initiations for two additional years. Figure 1 shows initiation rates through the childhood risk period plus two years. Initiation rates are based on those *entering each year of age without yet having committed the act in question.* (Otherwise we would have found a low rate of initiation to DRINK toward the end of childhood, just because most children were already drinking before then.)

Rates of school absence and failure were high in the first year of school, age six. Rates of onset of absence continued high at age seven and then declined rapidly, reaching close to zero by age 10. Children who did not fail their first two years of school also had rapidly decreasing risks of failure thereafter, reaching a low, steady level by age nine. Sex and alcohol use had very low rates of initiation through age 11, and then rapidly soaring rates that were still accelerating two years after our cut-off point (i.e., at age 16).

Arrests and dropouts both had low rates of initiation until age 13, and then began to rise. Dropouts peaked at 16, remained fairly high at 17 and then declined. Very few men were still at risk of dropout at 19 because by that age men had either already dropped out or had graduated from high school. Arrests rose through 15, remained steady through 17, and then declined. We investigated the possibility that this decline was due to entering the military, but we found that those who were *not* inducted also had a decline in arrest liability after 17.

Marijuana liability first became sizeable at 13, declined at 14, and then rose slowly. It had not peaked two years after the end of "childhood." Use of other drugs and alcohol problems began later, and rates of initiation remained virtually flat and close to zero. Leaving home began to climb after age 15 and marriage after age 16. Both rose steeply for two years and then declined slightly, presumably to rise again shortly.

In sum, for five behaviors, sex, alcohol, marijuana, leaving home, and marriage, rates of initiation were still high or climbing at the end of "childhood." Four of these five behaviors (all except marijuana) are clearly cases of "status" deviance, that is, behaviors that are expected of adults and treated as deviant only when done by children. Eventually every man in our sample had sexual experience, all but 2 percent drank, almost all left home and married. Eventually half the sample used marijuana, although only 20 percent had done so before 18. While the rising curve for marijuana might suggest that marijuana use, even though illegal, was also "status" deviance according to local standards, the rise in marijuana use was much less steep with the approach of adulthood than was the rise in other "status" deviant behaviors, suggesting that there are also pressures against marijuana use which, although stronger for younger than older persons, did not disappear with maturity.

The only behaviors for which the risk seemed to end spontaneously were the two elementary school behaviors (FAILURE and AB-SENCE) and ARREST. For all three, most onsets occurred within a narrow age span (six to seven for the school behaviors, 15 to 17 for ARREST), followed by a marked drop in rates thereafter. DROPOUT had the same pattern, but this was an artifact produced by graduation at ages 17 to 19.

The fact that hard-drug use did not follow marijuana's pattern of increasing risk with aging is particularly interesting, since, as we have shown in an earlier paper (Robins and Murphy, 1967), hard-drug use in this sample was almost always preceded by marijuana use. But we also showed in that paper that *early* marijuana users were at much greater risk of progression to hard drugs than those with later onset. The flat curves of hard-drug onsets show that the addition of new late onset users of marijuana was not reflected in corresponding increments in the use of other drugs, at least by age 19.

Ages with High Risk of Initiations

We have shown that different types of deviance tended to occur at different ages. By age five, only alcohol, sex, and arrest had occurred for any child. At age six, failing, dropout, and absence had been added for a total of six behaviors; at eight, the first children who left home or used marijuana appeared; and finally by 14, all 13 behaviors had occurred. The next year, the risk period for sex, alcohol, failure, and absence terminated, reducing the behaviors at risk to nine for the remainder of childhood.

On an average, the 223 men in our sample committed 3.2 types of deviance apiece, for a grand total of 707 acts. If onsets of these 707 acts were proportional to the number of behaviors at risk of onset, one would expect the curve of onsets by age to parallel the right-skewed stepped figure representing number of behaviors at risk

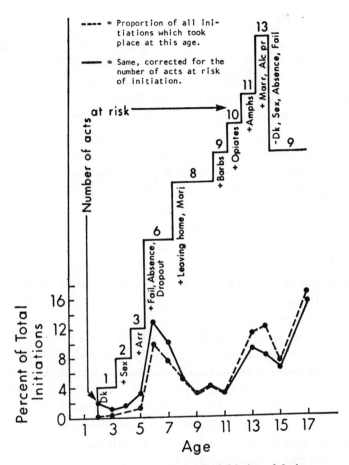

FIGURE 2. Ages with high risks for the initiation of deviance.

by age in Figure 2, and thus to reach a peak at age 14. Instead, when we looked to see at what ages the 707 deviant behaviors occurred, we found a trimodal curve of onsets (the dashed line in Figure 2) with peaks at age six, when 10 percent of all forms of deviance first occurred; at ages 13 and 14, when 11 and 12 percent of all deviant acts first occurred; and at age 17, when 17 percent of all deviant acts first occurred. Through age six, the curve of onsets follows the shape of the larger figure, reflecting the slow addition of opportunities for deviance before school entry and a sharp rise at school entry. After age 14 the curve declines, paralleling the end of risk periods for elementary school problems, sex, and alcohol. Between six and nine there is a decline in onsets of deviance and between 15 and 17 there is a rise, neither explained by the larger figure.

The dashed curve in Figure 2 shows the proportion of behaviors ever committed which were first committed at a particular age. It does not take into account either for how many acts that particular age fell into the risk period or how many children were still at risk of starting that behavior at that age because they had not done it earlier. To see whether the peak ages of risk shown by the dashed curve might not merely represent the effects of opportunities to commit acts rather than the true liability to new deviance at each age, we weighted the proportion of acts ever begun that began at a particular age by the fraction of total opportunities to begin that were available at that age. This correction resulted in the solid curve in Figure 2. This solid curve shows what the ages of highest risk of new deviance would have been if all the forms of deviant behavior had been available throughout childhood and if previous deviance had not reduced opportunities for new deviance. After this correction, the trimodal shape was preserved, although the second peak moved from age 14 to 13. We conclude, then, that there were three age periods at which the risk of initiating new forms of deviance was especially high—at school entry, at entering puberty (ages 13 and 14), and just before adulthood.

From our earlier observations (Figure 1) we understand the peak at age six to represent the tendency of elementary-school failure and absence to occur early if they occur at all, and the peak at 17 to represent the tendency for most other behaviors to cluster near the end of their risk periods. The decline after 14 may indicate a true temporary decline in the initiation of new forms of deviance shortly after puberty, but it may also be an artifact of our defining the beginning of the period of risk as the age at which the first member of the sample showed a particular behavior. Several rare forms of deviant behavior, marriage, alcohol problems, and amphetamine use, occurred in this sample for the first time at age 12 or 14. Thus at these ages the sample became "at risk" of a number of behaviors which very few children ever actually performed. Adding these behaviors to the denominator produced a drop in rate of initiations compar· able to the very low rate of initiations before school entry, when drinking, sex, and arrest were considered behaviors at risk because a few members of our sample reported their very early occurrence, although they seldom occurred so early.

Number of Deviant Acts per Child

On an average, men in our sample reported having committed (or their school and police records showed the commission of) 3.2 of the 13 behaviors we have considered. Figure 3 shows that the most common number of acts committed was one to three. As the number of acts increased, the number committing that many decreased. While no man committed all 13 of these acts, one did commit 12—he failed only to marry before age 18.

Is the Number of Deviant Acts Randomly Distributed?

In Figure 3, we find the distribution of number of different acts committed strongly skewed toward the left or lower end. A distribution skewed toward the left suggests a possible Poisson distribution. If we had a Poisson distribution, we would assume the variety of deviant acts was the result of a random process and there would be no need for any causal explanations, much less for positing a developmental model.

We tested the randomness of the distribution in two ways. When we tested it against the binomial distribution, assuming 13 independent trials, we got a highly significant difference ($t=4.14$, $p<.0001$). When we tested for goodness of fit to a Poisson distribution, we again found our results significantly different from expected values ($\chi^2=62.2$, $df=8$, $p<.0001$). As Figure 3 shows, our distribution has too many cases at both the lower and upper ends of the distribution to fit the Poisson model.

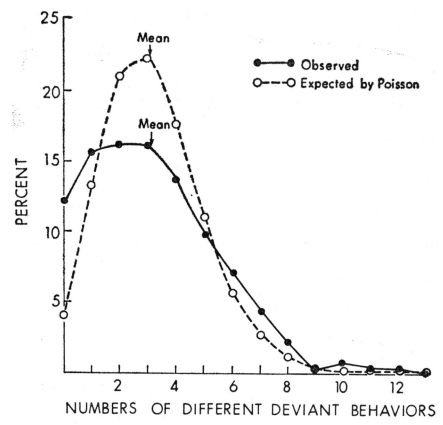

FIGURE 3.   Variety of deviant behavior in childhood.

Testing for the Occurrence of a Developmental Process

Having identified the commission of deviant behaviors as a non-random process, we have grounds for exploring whether there may not be a developmental process going on. There need not be, because the departure from randomness might be entirely explained by background variables (which have made some children relatively immune to deviance or others relatively deviance-prone or which have affected liability to *certain* of the behaviors we are investigating) or by effective interventions which affected only some children.

The present paper will not be able to *prove* that relationships we find between behaviors can be attributed to a developmental process, since we cannot rule out these other possibilities. However, we can describe the kind of relationships between acts we would expect to see if there *is* a developmental process at work, and learn to what extent the relationships found are consistent with such patterns.

A first expectation, if there is a developmental process, is that acts that are most common should be those that occur earliest in childhood. As a corollary, acts typically occurring late should imply the previous commission of many other acts. This follows from the fact that in a developmental process a later stage can be reached only after having passed through an earlier stage. A simple paradigm is that of height—where there are fewer people at least six feet tall than at least five feet tall and all six-footers have at some time passed every fixed increment in height between four and six feet, while five-footers have passed only half as many.

The expected relationships were indeed found. The rank-order correlation between an act's frequency rank (with the highest frequency equal to 1) and its rank by median age at initiation was —.70, and between its frequency rank and the number of other acts also committed was —.93. Thus rare acts occur late and imply the commission of many other acts.

A second expectation, if there is a developmental process, is that deviant acts should be intercorrelated, since if a later stage can be reached only by passing through an earlier one, any contingency table involving two acts that are part of that process will have one zero cell, for the case where the later act is positive and the earlier act is negative. Intercorrelations between pairs of behaviors were indeed common, positive, and strong (Table 2). Of the 78 2x2 contingency tables generated by 13 behaviors, 73 were positive and 42 (54 percent) were statistically significant and positive (p<.05, two-tailed), 21 times the number of significant positive relationships expected by chance. Indeed, 20 (26 percent) were significant at the p<.001 level, 513 times the number that should have been significant by chance. Every one of the 13 behaviors was significantly related to at least one other behavior.

TABLE 2

Significant Correlations between Behaviors

$p < .001$ (20)	ϕ	$p < .01$ (15)	ϕ
OPIATE-BARBS	.63	OP-ALP PR	.21
AMPH-BARBS	.46	DO-DK	.20
MJ-BARBS	.44	OP-ARR	.20
ALC PR-AMPH	.39	AMPH-DK	.20
FAIL-ABS	.39	MJ-DO	.19
OP-MJ	.38	MJ-ALC PR	.19
OP-AMPH	.37	DK-ALC PR	.19
DO-ABS	.33	ARR-ALC PR	.19
AMPH-MJ	.32	ABS-ARR	.19
LH-MARRY	.32	SEX-DO	.18
BARB-ALC PR	.30	MJ-LH	.17
DO-LH	.29	BARB-ARR	.17
DK-MJ	.29	BARB-LH	.17
SEX-MJ	.29	BARB-SEX	.17
DO-ARR	.27	OP-LH	.17
DO-FAIL	.24		
MJ-ARR	.23	$p < .05$ (7)	
DO-ALC PR	.22	OP-DO	.16
DK-LH	.22	ALC PR-SEX	.16
DK-SEX	.22	AMPH-ARR	.15
		DO-BARB	.13
		DK-BARB	.13
		ABS-LH	.13
		ABS-MARR	.13

A Quantitative vs. a Qualitative Process

While both quantitative and qualitative developmental processes imply correlations between deviant behaviors, *which* acts would be most strongly intercorrelated would differ. If the developmental process were entirely quantitative, so that committing any one act increased the likelihood of committing any other, *all* correlations between acts should be positive and the strength of correlation should depend primarily on *temporal* relationships. Earliest occurring acts (which are also the most frequent) should be most highly correlated with the next earliest and least strongly correlated with those appearing late (and rarest). If instead the causal relationships between acts were qualitative, one might expect some pairs of acts to be uncorrelated and one would expect strongest correlations between acts in the same conceptual realm, whether or not they occurred close to the same ages. That is, we would expect truancy to predict school dropout better than amphetamine use, even though amphetamine use is a bit closer to truancy in median age of first occurrence.

In examining the correlations between pairs of our 13 deviant behaviors, we found that not only were more than half positively correlated at a statistically significant level, but of the remainder, 31 of 36 were in the positive direction, and the five negative correlations were close to zero. While a quantitative developmental process would lead us to expect all relationships to be positive and, if the sample were of a reasonable size, all statistically significant, our failure to meet these criteria might be due only to too small a sample to show significant relationships when one of the pair of behaviors is rare. However, pairs of acts in which one or both behaviors were rare (occurring in less than 7 percent of the sample) were about as often significantly and positively correlated as pairs in which both acts were more common (52 percent vs. 57 percent). Thus, correlations seemed likely to be explainable at least in part by relationships between specific acts rather than all being part of one quantitative process.

Our second criterion for a purely quantitative developmental process was that acts adjacent in order of appearance should be the most strongly correlated. To see whether this criterion was met, we inquired whether the most highly correlated pairs of behaviors also had the smallest differences between the ranks of their median ages of initiation. There was a striking association between strength of correlation and similarity of ages of onset. When acts were especially strongly correlated ($p < .001$), the average difference between the ranks of their median age at initiation was 2.9. When the value of p was greater than .001 but less than .01, the average difference in ranks rose to 4.0, while for still less highly correlated pairs, it reached 5.7. On the other hand, the strongest correlations were also between acts that seemed conceptually related, a fact that would argue for a *qualitative* developmental process. The strongest relationships ($p < .001$) occurred between acts which both had to do with the use of mood-modifying drugs or which both represented school problems. Thus, while we have some evidence for a quantitative process, we also have grounds for suspecting that certain specific behaviors are likely to induce other specific behaviors.

However, to argue convincingly that certain specific behaviors caused others, we need to do more than show that correlations between acts from a similar conceptual realm were stronger than their similarity in frequency or age of onset could explain. We must also be able to show which behaviors were actually followed by others at a rate higher than chance expectation, and that these relationships were not spurious. The next section attacks this problem.

An Actuarial Test for Causal Relationships Between Specific Behaviors

To show in a nonexperimental setting that one specific type of act is a plausible cause of another specific act, one must begin with persons who have committed neither, and show that those who commit the first act (ACT 1) thereafter have an increased probability of committing the second (ACT 2). When the two acts share a common age-range of risk, the estimate of the change in probability attributable to the first act must be adjusted for the amount of risk period of the second act which had already elapsed before the occurrence of the first.

To make the requirement for adjusting for elapsed risk clear, let us assume that we want to see whether DROPOUT leads to AR-REST. Table 1 shows that dropouts occurred on the average at age 16.2, while arrests occurred at an average age of 15.2. Thus by the time the average dropout has occurred, most of the period at risk of arrest is already over. The only people in whom we can show a possible causal effect of dropout on arrest are those who dropped out *without* a prior arrest. This group not only typically had only a brief period still at risk of arrest after dropping out, but was made up of people who had not had early arrests. To compare arrests following dropout with the arrest rate of a comparable group who did not drop out, we must identify those persons who not only did not drop out, but who also survived without an arrest until the age at which the dropout left school. Only then will they have the same length of time at risk of arrest, the same age period at risk, and an equal resistance to early arrests.

To solve this problem we modified a classic age-adjusted actuarial method to manage a two-risk condition: the risk of the presumed cause (DROPOUT) and the risk of the presumed consequence (ARREST) (Robins and Taibleson, 1972). This method allows us to test the significance of a difference in rates of an effect between persons with and without a presumed cause, while instituting controls for age at risk of the effect.

All pairs of behaviors were tested by this method, when possible. Pairs were lost to testing (a) when the "cause" occurred too rarely (in less than ten persons) to allow confidence in the results (e.g., OPIATES and AMPH as causes provided no more than seven or nine cases, respectively, still at risk of any given other behavior), (b) when the "cause" occurred so late that no risk period for possible "effects" remained (e.g., since MARRIAGE generally occurred at age 17, there was no age of risk left for other behaviors to appear between its occurrence and our cut-off of childhood at 18), or (c) when the "effect" occurred so early that it inevitably preceded any possible "cause" (as FAIL could not be a consequence of DROPOUT). Of the 156 theoretically possible cause-effect pairs, given 13 behaviors, 84 could be tested.

Of 84 tests, 38 (45 percent) were statistically significant by chi-square test* (all those marked + in Table 3). Among the behaviors found to predict other behaviors, MARIJUANA, DROPOUT, and early DRINK were the most potent causes, predicting six or seven behaviors each, more than half of those for which tests were possible. DROPOUT and ALCOHOL PROBLEMS were the behaviors best predicted by other behaviors, each predicted by six of the other behaviors, all those in which tests were possible for DROPOUT

---

* There is no completely satisfactory way to test the significance of differences between age-adjusted rates for an additive two-risk model. Because of this problem, we have used an extremely conservative test, and may therefore be overlooking some causal relationships (see Robins and Taibleson, 1972).

TABLE 3

Results of Age-Adjusted Actuarial Tests and
Tests for Spuriousness

		MJ	DO	DK	BARB	CAUSES ARR	SEX	ABS	FAIL	LH
No. of Tests Possible as Cause:		9	8	11	2	12	12	12	12	6
EFFECTS	No. of Tests Possible as Effect:									
DO	6	+		+*		+*	+*	+**	+*	
ALCP	9	+	+*	+*	+	+	+	0	0	0
BARB	7	+*	+	0		+	+*	0	0	
LH	7	+	+*	+**		0	0	+**	0	
ARR	7	+*	+	0			0	+*	0	0
MJ	7		+.	+**		0	+*	0	0	0
DK	5	0				+*	+*	0	0	
OP	8	+*	+*	0		+	0	0	0	0
AMPH	8	+*	0	+**		0	0	0	0	+
ABS	3					0	0		+**	
FAIL	4		0			0	0	+**		
SEX	4		+*			0		0	0	
MARR	9	0	0	0	0	0	0	+**	0	0

+ = p<.06 by actuarial test before controls to check spuriousness.
0 = p>.06
Relationships that were not testable are left blank.
 * Controlling on significant predictors of cause and effect, if any, did not reduce to n.s.
** Controlling on both predictors and number of prior behaviors did not reduce to n.s.

(that is, not blank in the DROPOUT row of Table 3), and two-thirds of possible tests for ALCOHOL PROBLEMS.

Tests for Spuriousness

The age-adjusted method described thus far has not considered the possible spuriousness of these relationships. When an event has multiple significant "causes" (as DROPOUT, for instance, is predicted by six different behaviors), some of these "causes" may be the effects of other of these "causes," and simply happen to occur at a younger age than the event of interest. To see whether a causal relationship has been spuriously attributed, it is usual to hold constant any variables preceding and correlated with both the imputed cause and the imputed outcome. If the correlation between the "cause" and "effect" then remains significant, one assumes that the common precursor has not engendered a spurious relationship, and that the causal relationship remains plausible.

In the present study there remains one problem, however. Even after we control on a correlated behavior, the "with cause" group necessarily has on the average at least one more deviant behavior while still at risk of the "effect" than does the group of matched controls, because it has the "cause" itself. And if that cause is also correlated with other forms of deviance *not* correlated with our effect and therefore not held constant, the "with cause" group may easily exceed the "without cause" group in average number of prior deviant behaviors by more than one. Then, if there is a quantitative developmental process, that is, if more deviant behaviors in the past mean a greater risk of some new type of deviance, we may find the "cause" significantly predicting our "effect" even if there is no real specific causal relationship between them. Because both specific behaviors and number of previous behaviors can create spurious relationships, we instituted controls for both types of spuriousness.

Controlling on Specific Precursors

To test for spuriousness due to some third form of deviant behavior's explaining both the "cause" and the "effect," we selected a matched "without cause" case for every "with cause" case, while controlling on the presence or absence of any third type of deviance that had been found to significantly predict both the "cause" and its "effect." We then tested for a significantly higher proportion showing the "effect" after the "cause" than in its absence.

A "without cause" case was defined as an appropriate match for a "with cause" case if it met three conditions: (1) the "causal" behavior either did not occur before 18 (or before 15 for sex and alcohol) or occurred only after the behavior thought to be its "effect" had already occurred; (2) the "without cause" child had reached the age at which the child "with cause" first demonstrated the "causal" behavior without yet having committed the "effect" behavior; (3) if the "with cause" child had already shown the third form of deviant behavior that might render the "cause" spurious by the age he first showed the "cause," the "without cause" child had also shown it by that age, and if the "with cause" child had not shown that third type of behavior by that age, the "without cause" child also had not.

The first criterion identified the potential match as "without cause," the second criterion guaranteed an identical age period at risk of the "effect," and the third criterion guaranteed that the cases matched with respect to the presence or absence of a third variable that might render the cause-effect relationship spurious.

As an example, to test whether the finding that DROPOUT leads to ARREST was spurious, we controlled successively on the two events found significant predictors of both: ABSENCE and MARIJUANA (note that these are the only two variables with a + in both the DROPOUT and ARREST rows in Table 3). Suppose that when controlling on MARIJUANA, we found that our first "with cause" case had dropped out at 14 and had first smoked marijuana at age 13. From the randomly ordered data set, the next case was selected as his match who either never dropped out or did so only after arrest (i.e., was not a dropout when arrested, if arrested), who had not been arrested before or at 14, and who had used marijuana by age 14. Therefore, the matched "without cause" case had never been simultaneously a dropout and at risk of arrest; he was at risk of arrest during the same age period (15 to 17) as the dropout; and, like the dropout, he had used marijuana prior to this risk period. When a match could not be found, the "with cause" case was dropped. The loss of cases resulting from dropping unmatched cases made finding significant results more difficult. Not only were there fewer cases in which to test significance, but those lost were disproportionately cases in which there was an early cause plus a precursor, since these were the most difficult to match. These lost cases were the very cases at greatest risk of the effect, since they had more precursors and a longer period at risk. Losing them reduced the proportion of affected cases in the sample, thus reducing the chance of showing a significant relationship.

McNemar's test for matched pairs was applied to see whether the cause-effect relationship had survived this test for spuriousness. A cause-effect relationship was considered to have survived if the number of "with cause" cases showing the outcome still significantly ($p < .11$) exceeded the number of "without cause" cases showing it.

In Table 3 where there are one or two asterisks, relationships initially found significant by the actuarial method have survived all these tests for spuriousness. (Note that DROPOUT no longer predicted ARREST when ABSENCE and MARIJUANA were held constant.) Eleven of the relationships we had found by actuarial methods had no significant precursor of both events, and therefore no test for spuriousness was necessary. Of the remaining 27 relationships significant by the actuarial method and tested for spuriousness, 15 survived, despite our having had to discard unmatched cases. Among the survivors, DRINK was the most frequent predictor of other forms of deviance, predicting six other types. MARIJUANA and ABSENCE each predicted five other behaviors. DROPOUT was the behavior most susceptible to the influence of other behaviors. It was predicted by five different behaviors: FAIL, ABSENCE, DRINK, SEX, and ARREST. No other behavior had more than three predictors shown to be nonspurious. All 13 types of deviant behaviors survived this first set of tests for spuriousness as an effect of some other form of deviance, and seven behaviors survived as a cause as well: ABSENCE, FAIL, DRINK, SEX, ARREST, MARIJUANA, and DROPOUT.

Controlling on the Number of Prior Deviant Behaviors

To see whether the causal relationships that withstood the test of holding constant the predictors of both cause and effect would also withstand the test of holding constant the number of previous behaviors, we again found matches among the "without cause" cases for the "with cause" cases. Cases were defined as "with" and "without" cause just as they were in our first test for spuriousness, and the cases were put into random order as before. Again the first matching case was selected, but the qualification for matching was now the number of previous behaviors rather than the type. A matching "without cause" case in this test was required to have exactly the same number of deviant behaviors through the age at which the "cause" first occurred as did the "with cause" case. Since the "cause" was itself a deviant behavior, the "without cause" case was required to have the same number of other forms of deviance as the "with cause" case plus one more to make up for the absent "cause." No attention was paid to whether or not the types of deviance were the same. When SEX or DRINK occurred beyond age 15, they were ignored—that is, they were not counted as deviant behaviors. Again cases were discarded when no match could be found, and again those unmatchable were cases at the greatest risk of the outcome—those with the largest number of precursors.

The 26 relationships that survived the test for controlling for specific precursors were now tested to see whether it might be the *number* of earlier behaviors rather than the presumed "cause" that predicted the later behavior. Only eight of these relationships survived this second test at a statistically significant level. These successful survivors are marked with double asterisks in Table 3. The eight surviving relationships included as causes early drinking, which increased the risk of marijuana and amphetamine use, and excessive elementary-school absence, which led to failure in elementary school, dropout from high school, early marriage, and leaving home before 18. Additionally, failure in elementary school led to excessive absence, these two elementary-school forms of deviance thus having a reciprocal relationship.

Even when results were not statistically significant, in all but four cases (DRINK and SEX as causes of each other and of DROPOUT) the outcome occurred more often when the presumed cause was among the preceding deviant behaviors than when it was absent from the same number of preceding deviant behaviors. For nine of these nonsignificant relationships, the proportion of cases in which the effect occurred was at least half again as large following the "cause" than in its absence, but with an equally extensive prior history of deviance. Relationships that approached significance after both tests for spuriousness had been applied included as causes DRINK and DROPOUT, both of which portended ALCOHOL PROBLEMS, and ARRESTS, which led to drinking before 14. Early SEX experience predicted MARIJUANA use, which in turn predicted use of all other types of illicit drugs as well as juvenile ARREST. The use of OPIATES was additionally predicted by high-school DROPOUT.

Given these trends even in the absence of many statistically significant results, it seems probable that most of our possible "causes" actually were making some contribution to these "effects," although the sharp drop in the number of significant relationships when the number of prior behaviors was held constant provides further evidence that the developmental process was in part a quantitative one.

How Important Are These Specific Acts as "Causes"?

The fact that one act apparently increased the risk of another does not necessarily mean that this effect had practical importance. Table 4 evaluates the importance of every relationship between pairs of behaviors that was shown statistically significant by age-adjusted actuarial test and continued to be significant after controlling on precursors common to the pair, and which was still at or near significance after holding constant the number of prior types of deviance.

How important it is to know that one act leads to another depends in part on whether that first act is either a necessary or sufficient cause of the second. The first act approximates a necessary cause if the second act almost never occurs unless preceded by the first; it approximates a sufficient cause if the first act is almost invariably followed by the second. (Of course, from a purely practical point of view, necessary and sufficient causes which cannot be controlled are less important than less powerful causes that are subject to control. Other things being equal, however, the potential for control is greatest when the cause is necessary or sufficient.)

TABLE 4

Were Any Acts Necessary or Sufficient Causes of Others?

	NECESSARY? How Often Was the Second Act Preceded by the First?	SUFFICIENT? How Often Was the First Act Followed by the Second?
"NECESSARY"	%	%
MARJ→OPIATE	92	15
DRINK→AMPH	85	10
SEX→MARJ	78	25
DRINK→ALC PROB	76	12
DROPOUT→OPIATE	75	8
MARJ→BARB	59	14
"SUFFICIENT"		
ARREST→DRINK	21	51
MARJ→ARREST	16	36
BOTH (?)		
ABSENCE→DROPOUT	60	54
DRINK→LEAVE HOME	58	44
ABSENCE→LEAVE HOME	55	33

None of the "causal" behaviors in Table 4 seemed *sufficient* to produce further types of deviance. The closest approximations to sufficient causes were ABSENCE in elementary school, which half the time was followed by school DROPOUT, and ARREST in children who had not yet begun to drink, which was followed by early DRINKING in half the cases. In only two other relationships, ABSENCE as a cause of LEAVING HOME and MARIJUANA as a cause of ARREST, did the "effect" actually occur in even one-third of the cases at risk following the "cause." Thus, if our findings were used to select children for intervention on the basis of their having committed a form of deviance likely to lead to more serious behavior, many children would be selected who would not actually commit the predicted deviance even if no intervention took place (or who would commit it only later, in adulthood).

While there are few sufficient causes in our list, there are a number of examples among our deviant behaviors for which an earlier type of deviance appears virtually necessary. The two most striking examples are both forms of illicit drug use. OPIATES were used almost solely by children who had already used MARIJUANA (92 percent), even though very few marijuana users (15 percent) went on to use opiates while they were still children. Opiate users were also almost always (75 percent) previously high school DROPOUTS, although again only 8 percent of dropouts went on to use opiates before their eighteenth birthdays. The use of AMPHETAMINES occurred almost exclusively (85 percent) among children who had begun DRINKING before 15, as did ALCOHOL PROBLEMS before 18 (76 percent). MARIJUANA use was largely restricted (78 percent) to children who had already had SEX experience. (The fact that MARIJUANA use is a virtual prerequisite for OPIATE use has been noted in a number of studies (Kandel, 1975). The association of amphetamine use with early drinking has not been so commonly observed.)

When a cause of a selected behavior is sufficient but not necessary, preventing the occurrence of that cause may reduce the total number of cases of the behavior of interest only slightly. When the cause of a selected behavior is necessary but not sufficient, preventing the occurrence of the cause will wipe out all cases of the behavior, but only at the cost of interfering with the lives of many people who would never have shown the behavior even if we had not intervened. When a cause is both necessary and sufficient, we need have less concern about unwarranted intervention and can have greater optimism about achieving our goals. We have three relationships that approach this highly desirable situation: elementary school absence (truancy) leading to high-school dropout and premature departure from home, and drinking before 15 also leading to premature departure from home. If there is a practical message in our efforts, it is that centering our preventive efforts on school attendance and early drinking is likely to have the greatest payoff at least cost.

More Complex Sequences of Causation

We have discovered a set of pairs of temporally ordered, nonspurious relationships that argue for specific influences between different types of deviance. If acts are linked in cause-effect pairs, it is possible that these pairs are themselves organized into longer causal chains, the simplest of which is A→B→C, where A has been shown to cause B, and B to cause C. Exploring such simple chains provides an opportunity to see to what degree the development of deviant behaviors approaches a Markov process, in which the link between B and C in the A→B→C chain should be no stronger than were the chain $\overline{A}$→B→C, that is, where B occurred without A.

An examination of Table 4 shows a large number of logically possible chains that could be generated by hooking together pairs of temporally ordered cause-effect relationships. The patterns so generated are shown in Figure 4. The numbers above the arrows in Figure 4 refer to the 17 triads that appear in these sequences.

An effort to explore the Markovian properties of these triads in our current sample foundered on our sample size, given the need to discard cases where any two of the three events occurred at the same age (because the order was then unknown), the short spans of risk, and the fact that we could identify a three-event sequence only if the three acts occurred in the required sequence, with each act occurring at a different age. Of the 17 triads in Figure 4, there are only two in which at least 20 cases experienced both the sequences A→B and $\overline{A}$→B while still at risk of C. In both triads the A→B variables were ABSENCE→DROPOUT. The two "Cs" were OPIATES and ALCOHOL PROBLEMS. In examining these two triads, we found no reason to discard the Markovian model since rates of the third variable were very similar whether the DROPOUT occurred after ABSENCE or without it. (Under both circumstances 9 percent used OPIATES; 11 percent later developed ALCOHOL PROBLEMS if DROPOUT had been preceded by ABSENCE, and 13 percent when it had not.)

DISCUSSION

Our excursion into the study of the development of deviance in the childhoods of young, urban-born, black men reviewed the frequency, ages at initiation, and temporal patterning of 13 forms of

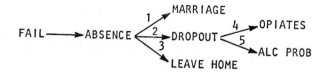

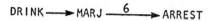

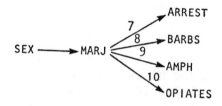

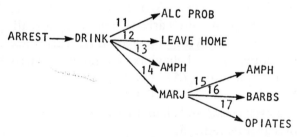

Figure 4. Possible chains of causation among deviant behaviors.

deviance. Vulnerability to beginning new kinds of deviance was found highest at ages 6, 13, 14, and 17. All 13 types of deviance were found to be linked statistically into a common network. Those behaviors beginning young were the most common and the most likely to occur alone. The patterning of deviance was not a random process. There were more highly deviant and more nondeviant children than would have been expected by chance. This set us looking to see whether there might be a developmental process at work.

Evidence supporting a developmental process included the facts that the most frequently committed acts were those committed young, there were strong correlations between pairs of behaviors, and the strongest correlations were between pairs of behaviors initiated at about the same age and conceptually related. These findings suggested a developmental process made up of both quantitative and qualitative relationships.

Qualitative relationships were tested by an age-adjusted actuarial method followed by tests for spuriousness which required holding constant acts that were presumptive causes of both members of a pair of acts as well as the total number of prior acts. A few relationships survived these tests. Failure in elementary school did lead to serious school absence and vice versa. Excessive school absence predicted dropout, leaving the family home before 18, and early marriage. Early drinking (before 15) predicted use of marijuana and amphetamines and leaving home before 18. In addition, there were nine relationships close to significance, in which early drinking, early sex, marijuana use, arrests, and dropout all predicted later forms of deviance. While none of these early behaviors was *sufficient* to produce other behaviors, several were virtually *necessary*. Three relationships (ABSENCE→DROPOUT, DRINK→ LEFT HOME, ABSENCE→LEFT HOME) came close enough to being both necessary *and* sufficient to make them attractive candidates for efforts at intervention.

In addition to these specific relationships, the fact that many relationships between specific pairs of behaviors were reduced by controlling on number of prior acts suggests that the development of deviance in childhood also has an important quantitative aspect. It may be that the more varied the prior experience with deviant behavior, the greater becomes the readiness to commit still other types of deviance. If this is so, we can reliably forecast who will experiment with new forms of deviance—the pioneers will be those who already have a broad experience in "conventional" deviant behaviors.

The relationships that we have found among diverse forms of deviance in childhood are consistent with believing that deviance, like growth, has a developmental aspect, but they do not prove it. These relationships among behaviors could also occur simply because family and other background factors produce more than one form of deviance and thus account for the intercorrelations between these various forms. Further analysis going outside the patterning of the acts themselves to hold constant background causes will be needed to take this argument further. Meanwhile, the present analysis has pinpointed relationships between deviant behaviors that are prime candidates for further exploration.

In our efforts to establish the plausibility of a developmental process, a number of requirements had to be met. We needed to know not only what behaviors had occurred but in what order and at what ages. We needed to consider whether children at the time they first performed the behavior that might contribute to the appearance of some subsequent form of deviance had not already passed at least some of the age of risk of developing the second type. If so, the real effects could have been hidden unless the comparison group had been limited to other children at the same stage. When one form of deviance was shown to lead to another with a statistically significant frequency, two sources of spuriousness had to be investigated—first, that some other behavior may have caused both, and second, that it was just the fact that *some* deviant behavior had occurred first, rather than a specific effect of the first behavior, which accounted for the increased risk.

Our data were sometimes inadequate to handle all these requirements simultaneously. One would have liked a larger and less homogeneous sample of children followed prospectively via a panel design. Such a sample could have been asked yearly or more frequently about the appearance during the last interval of any behaviors still absent at the last inquiry, and about their order of appearance if more than one type had been initiated. A large prospective study of this kind would not only produce more reliable results than did our small retrospective one, but would allow for the exploration of questions for which our data were too incomplete or too scattered:

(a) does the *severity* of the deviance matter? (b) Does the age at which it first occurs matter? (c) Are there common extended chains that involve multiple types of deviant behaviors? (d) Does the developmental pattern replicate across sex, race, and class groups?

Our own efforts have only scratched the surface, but they have been encouraging in indicating that there seems to be a process to be studied. If we begin to understand deviance as a developmental process, we will begin to know how to select children at high risk of later problems and *what* problems we should try to protect them from.

REFERENCES

KANDEL, D. 1975. Stages in adolescent involvement in drug use. *Science,* 190:912-914.

ROBINS, L. N. 1966. *Deviant Children Grown Up: Sociological and Psychiatric Study of Sociopathic Personality.* Baltimore: Williams & Wilkins. Reprinted 1974, Huntington, N.Y.: Robert E. Krieger.

ROBINS, L. N., and MURPHY, G. E. 1967. Drug use in a normal population of young Negro men. *Am. J. Public Health,* 57:1580-1596.

ROBINS, L. N., MURPHY, G. E., and BRECKENRIDGE, M. B. 1968. Drinking behavior of young Negro men. *Q. J. Stud. Alcohol,* 29:657-684.

ROBINS, L. N., MURPHY, G. E., WOODRUFF, R. A., JR., and KING, L. J. 1971. The adult psychiatric status of black school boys. *Arch. Gen. Psychiatry,* 24:338-345.

ROBINS, L. N., and TAIBLESON, M. H. 1972. An actuarial method for assessing the direction of influence between two datable life events. *Sociological Methods and Research,* 1:243-270.

14

Sex- and Gender-Role Identification: The Sociobiological Process

RICHARD GREEN, M.D.

Research into sex- and gender-role identification in children has become increasingly complex. New and more sophisticated strategies have been introduced and larger numbers of qualified investigators have entered the field. Amid this surge of research energy has also appeared politicization in response to the question, "How do children develop a sexual identity?" This paper will highlight some of the research strategies of contemporary investigators in developmental psychology, psychoanalysis, human ethology, neuroendocrinology, nonhuman primate ethology, clinical psychology, and psychiatry. It will also focus on the areas engulfed by political controversy.

PRENATAL INFLUENCES

Research is progressing with increased vigor into possible prenatal influences on postnatal sex-typed behaviors. The discovery, over a decade ago, that exposing the female rhesus monkey fetus to high levels of male hormone produced male-type behavior after birth (a result not produced by *post*natal exposure to androgen), brought into focus a new area of inquiry into sexual development (Young, Goy, and Phoenix, 1964). Is the developing brain organized by sex-steroids in a male or female direction as are the reproductive structures?

The obvious human parallel to the laboratory experiment is the

257

virilizing adrenogenital syndrome in the female. Here the fetus is also exposed to unusually high levels of androgen which are produced by the fetus as a result of an inborn error of metabolism. The source of androgen in this case, in contrast to the monkey experiment in which androgen was introduced to the fetus via injections, is an experiment of nature. Studies of female children with the adrenogenital syndrome suggest that they participate more in rough-and-tumble and sports play, and show less interest in doll play and in bearing children. They are more often called "tomboys" (Ehrhardt and Baker, 1974).

Research in the human male is less convincing. One study suggested that both six- and 16-year-old males exposed prenatally to exogenously administered estrogen and progesterone (female hormones) were less rough-and-tumble and aggressive than a contrast group of males not exposed to hormones (Yalom, Green, and Fisk, 1973). Additionally, a few males with Kleinfelter's syndrome, who have deficient testes and low testosterone (androgen) levels, have appeared at clinics requesting sex-reassignment surgery to female status (Baker and Stoller, 1968; Money and Pollitt, 1964). One interpretation of the concurrence of Kleinfelter's syndrome and transsexualism in the same individual is the lower prenatal level of androgen reaching the developing central nervous system.

Assuming that prenatal levels of androgen have the effect of organizing the developing nervous system so that various types of behavior are more likely to become manifest, what effect might this have on sex-role socialization? Consider the behaviors at issue: rough-and-tumble, aggressive, and doll play. In our culture, these behaviors have sex-typed connotations. The male child disinclined to rough-and-tumble and sports play, but preferring doll play, will have a different peer-group socialization experience and a different mother-child and father-child relationship. Dramatic examples of such children will be described later. Conversely, girls disinclined to play with dolls and oriented primarily toward sports and rough-house play will also experience a different early-life socialization process than those preoccupied with frilly dresses and Barbie dolls (Green, 1976).

NEONATAL INFLUENCES

Researchers have spent considerable time and effort in mother-and-baby watching during the infant's first weeks and months of life in an attempt to discover differential manners by which male and female infants are treated by their primary caretaker. Although this research has yielded some statistically significant differences with respect to the amount of touching, style of touching, and degree of vocalization, considerable intrasex differences remain, and there is no compelling synthesis of just how these differences mold sexual identity or gender-role behavior. The above notwithstanding, it does appear that human males, by the second half of the first year, are more autonomous with respect to their mothers, spending less time in physical and visual contact with them (Lewis and Weinraub, 1974). There is also evidence that, by the end of the first year, sex differences in play style exist as do differences in reaction to frustration (Goldberg and Lewis, 1969). These differences too are supported by parallel findings in nonhuman primate research (Rosenblum, 1974).

One neonatal sex difference that has been replicated is the prone head reaction. Newborn males placed on their abdomen are better able to raise their heads from the horizontal position (Bell and Costello, 1964). This suggests a greater degree of gross motor development, believed to be the result of high levels of prenatal androgen. The clinical question is: When does this intersex difference become developmentally and socially significant for the given individual? While no one would question that, as a population, adult males have greater strength and athletic skills than females (note Olympic records), significant intrasex differences exist. However, the age at which these differences emerge in a socially significant manner has not been fully clarified.

By the end of the second year of life, children appear to have a basic self-concept of being male or female (Green, 1976; Money, Hampson, and Hampson, 1955; Stoller, 1968). Provocative evidence exists that 13-month-old children can discriminate same-age children of the same sex from those of the other sex (Lewis and Weinraub,

1974). A series of pictures of 13- to 18-month-old male and female infants, with only facial features visible, were first shown to a group of adults and then to same-age infants. The adults were unable to discriminate the sex of the infants in the picture any better than by chance. However, infants spent more time looking at pictures of their own sex. In another study, the same investigators placed four children, two boys and two girls, into a rectangular enclosure. Each child was permitted, in turn, to crawl toward one of the other three children. The odds of crawling to an opposite-sex child are two to one, yet the majority of children crawled toward a same-sex infant.

Thus, there seems to be some capacity for same- and other-sex discrimination at the end of the first year which may be the initial component in establishing core-morphologic sexual identity (the self-concept of being male or female). This is not to say that this process is entirely innate. Parents respond to and rear male and female infants differently. From the moment of birth, whether it be the color of clothing and bedding, behavioral expectations, or toys, a dimorphic sex-typed socialization process begins.

Some parents protest against the traditional sex-typing of children and are attempting to raise their child in a more unigendered manner. The extent to which such child-rearing practices will "take" remains to be seen. Children are exposed to multiple socialization influences, not merely those presented by their parents. Thus, a child is also exposed to mass-media, peer-group influences, parents of the peer group, and the school socialization process. Studies of children in various types of early school settings and those raised by parents with divergent attitudes toward sex-typed child-rearing practices may clarify the degree to which traditional early gender-role behavior is modifiable. And, if modifiable, to what extent will it endure?

ATYPICAL SEX-ROLE DEVELOPMENT IN CHILDREN

Our principal research during the past decade has focused on grade school-age children showing atypical gender-role behavior. We have been studying children who prefer the toys, games, activities, dress, and companionship of other-sex children. Role-playing is typically as children or adults of the other sex. The children state their wish to be of the other sex.

Our earlier research focused on male children for several reasons. The first consideration was the retrospectively recalled childhood histories given by adults with an atypical sexual identity. Transsexuals (males requesting surgical and hormonal sex-reassignment to female status) universally recall their childhood as characterized by a compelling preference for the games, clothing, and activities of girls (Benjamin, 1966; Green and Money, 1969). In a series of 500 transvestites (adult males who fetishistically cross-dress) about half recalled the onset of their cross-dressing as having occurred during the preadolescent years (Prince and Bentler, 1972). In a study of about 150 male homosexuals and heterosexuals (Saghir and Robins, 1973), two-thirds of the male homosexual adults (significantly more than the heterosexual group) recalled a "girl-like" syndrome during childhood. Furthermore, the number of anatomic males requesting surgical sex-change is about three times that of females requesting sex-change (Green and Money, 1969); there are essentially no female transvestites (Stoller, 1968), and there are probably twice as many male as female homosexuals (Kinsey, Pomeroy, and Martin, 1948; Kinsey et al., 1953). Finally, there are many more atypical young females ("tomboys") than atypical males ("sissies"). Thus the probability that a young male who manifests cross-sex behavior will emerge into an adult with an atypical sexual identity is greater than that of the atypical young female. (And, since feminine behavior in boys results in social ostracism and conflict in the child and parents, it is more likely that "sissies" will be referred to a clinic than will "tomboys" whose behavior is generally accepted and nonconflictual.)

Our sample consisted of 60 males initially evaluated between age four and eleven who preferred dressing in girls' clothing, played with Barbie dolls as their favorite toy, typically role-played as a female in house games, typically imitated female characters from books, movies, and television, had a female peer group, avoided rough-and-tumble play and sports, and stated their wish to be girls. These children were evaluated by direct observation, psychological testing, and clinical interviewing. Transcripts of interviews with these children have been reported (Green, 1974). Their parents were extensively interviewed and tested. Excerpts of interviews with the parents have also been published (Green, 1974). A control group of same-age boys manifesting typical sex-typed behavior was gathered. Fifty families were matched for age of the child, sibling sequence, marital configuration of the family, ethnic background, and educational level of the father. Details of the demographic matching and behavioral contrasts of the two samples of boys and some preliminary data on the parents may be found in Green (1976).

More recently we have gathered a sample of "tomboys." Within the same age range as the boys, these are girls who do not play with female-type dolls, prefer rough-and-tumble athletic play (primarily with boys), prefer boys as playmates, insist on wearing masculine clothing, role-play as a male most of the time, and have stated their wish to be boys. They are considered to be "tomboys" by their parents. These children and their parents are undergoing psychological testing and clinical interviewing like the two family groups described above. We are currently collecting a control group of same-age girls who behave in a more stereotypically feminine manner, matching the two groups like the previously described male samples. Our study goal is to follow the four samples into adolescence and to correlate emerging and, ultimately, adult patterns of sexual identity with early patterns of gender-role behavior, parental characteristics, and family socialization influences.

CHILDREN OF THE SEXUALLY ATYPICAL

Another strategy in our attempts to better understand the processes of psychosexual development is a study of children being raised by adults whose sexual identity is atypical. These are the children being raised by transsexual or homosexual parents. As more persons undergo sex-reassignment procedures and either adopt children, become parents through donor insemination, or marry partners with children from a previous marriage, the number of children being raised by transsexuals increases. In such cases two parents were born as persons of the same sex although one now appears as a person of the opposite sex.

During the past year we have evaluated 14 children being raised in families in which one parent is transsexual. Seven are being raised by female-to-female transsexuals and seven by male-to-female transsexuals. Their age range is 13 to 20. They have lived in the transsexual household for one to 14 years.

The most remarkable socialization experience of the group is one in which four girls watched their biological mother evolve into their legal father. The parent had received androgen injections and a series of female-to-male surgical procedures. The children ranged in age from four to ten as the transition process began and are now between 13 and 20. Remarried, the biological parent is now in the role of husband to the children's "stepmother." These female children all have a basic female identity, are feminine in behavior, and exclusively heterosexual. To date, all 14 children show an appropriate core-morphologic gender identity, have typical sex-typed play preferences and vocational goals, and for those who have evolved sexual interests, are heterosexual.

In the households with homosexual mothers, 21 children have been evaluated. The evaluations occurred during court litigation involving child custody. All of the children have lived with their lesbian mothers and the mothers' female companion. The number of years in which the children have lived in these households ranges from two to six years. The age range of the children is five to 14. Eleven are male and ten are female. To date, all of the children show an appropriate core-morphologic sexual identity, typical sex-typed play behaviors, have typical sex-typed vocational goals, and look forward to conventional heterosexual families during adulthood.

Clearly, having a transsexual or homosexual parent poses a series of intriguing questions with respect to psychosexual development. Many influences on the sex-typing process may be postulated, based either on psychoanalytic or social-learning theory. To date, however, the children who have been evaluated seem to be developing typical psychosexual patterns. These children will be followed for comprehensive assessment of their development. In addition, a more systematic study with a control sample is being generated to better assess the influence of parental sexual orientation and sexual identity per se on the psychological development of children.

ETHICAL ISSUES

Because of the long-overdue arrival of increased public sensitivity to the sexism extant in our culture, as well as the discrimination experienced by persons with atypical sexual life-styles, much of the research described above has engaged controversy. There are those who believe that no innate sex differences exist, and that all documented behavioral differences are purely the product of socialization. There are those who believe that the great similarity in sex differences at the cross-cultural level points to biological imperatives that lead to the sex-typed behaviors seen and that these are not cross-cultural accidents. The compromisers in the field seek an accommodation between these two polarized viewpoints. They suggest an interface between innate differences in behavior, which in a cultural context imparts to them sex-typed implications, and thus has an effect on socialization. (One example would be a boy with low prenatal androgen levels who likes to play with a Barbie doll.)

Others strongly object to the study of children with atypical sex-typed behavioral patterns, charging that such research is nothing more than an effort to find causes of "deviant" adult behaviors and thus to eliminate an alternate sexual life-style. Others, equally convinced of the merit of their position, assert that "alternate sexual life-style" is nothing more than a euphemism for perversion, that the genesis of these behaviors should be discovered, and that children with such behaviors should be treated during childhood to prevent their later emergence. The moderates express concern for the immediate conflict experienced by the atypical male child in consequence of his very feminine behavior in a culture that continues to stigmatize such behavior. Those with this concern attempt to reduce the immediate conflict by some broadening of the child's behavioral base. They contend that if they can make the child happier, currently, this is a service to the child and family, and that if they can prevent the more extreme patterns of later atypical sexual identity, such as transsexualism, they will prevent subsequent conflict as well (Green, 1974).

Conclusion

Sexual identity is a basic personality component. Sexual identity affects us all. Much remains to be learned about how we become male or female, masculine and/or feminine, heterosexual, homosexual, or ambisexual. Much remains to be done with respect to providing an equal opportunity for a conflict-free developmental process for persons whose sex-typed behaviors do not fit historically conventional standards. We have responsibilities as researchers not to neglect the social implications of our work and the manner by which we can be of value on the larger public scale. At the same time, as scientists, we also have a responsibility to discover just how we become *who* we are, and *when*.

REFERENCES

Baker, H., and Stoller, R. 1968. Can a biological force contribute to gender identity? *Am. J. Psychiatry*, 124:1653-1658.

Bell, R., and Costello, N. 1964. Three tests for sex differences in tactile sensitivity in the newborn. *Biol. Neonatology*, 7:335-347.

Benjamin, H. 1966. *The Transsexual Phenomenon.* New York: Julian Press.

Ehrhardt, A., and Baker, S. 1974. Fetal androgens, human central nervous system differentiation, and behavior sex differences. In R. Friedman, R. Richart, and R. Van de Wiele (eds.), *Sex Differences in Behavior*, pp. 33-52. New York: Wiley.

Goldberg, S., and Lewis, M. 1969. Play behavior in the year old infant—early sex differences. *Child Dev.*, 40:21-31.

Green, R. 1974. *Sexual Identity Conflict in Children and Adults.* New York: Basic Books. Baltimore: Penguin.

Green, R. 1976. One-hundred-ten feminine and masculine boys: Behavioral contrasts and demographic similarities. *Arch. Sex. Behav.* 5:425-446.

Green, R., and Money, J. (eds.), 1969. *Transsexualism and Sex Reassignment.* Baltimore: Johns Hopkins Press.

Kinsey, A., Pomeroy, W., and Martin, C. 1948. *Sexual Behavior in the Human Male.* Philadelphia: Saunders.

Kinsey, A., Pomeroy, W., Martin, C., and Gebhard, P. 1953. *Sexual Behavior in the Human Female.* Philadelphia: Saunders.

Lewis, M., and Weinraub, M. 1974. Sex of parent x sex of child: Socioemotional development. In R. Friedman, R. Richart, and R. Van de Wiele (eds.), *Sex Differences in Behavior*, pp. 165-190. New York: Wiley.

MONEY, J., HAMPSON, J., and HAMPSON, J. 1955. An examination of some basic sexual concepts: The evidence of human hermaphroditism. *Bulletin of The Johns Hopkins Hospital*, 97:301-319.

MONEY, J., and POLLITT, E. 1964. Cytogenetic and psychosexual ambiguity. *Arch. Gen. Psychiatry*, 11:589-595.

PRINCE, C., and BENTLER, P. 1972. Survey of 504 cases of transvestism. *Psychol. Rep.*, 31:903-917.

ROSENBLUM, L. 1974. Sex differences, environmental complexity, and mother-infant interaction. *Arch. Sex. Behav.*, 3:117-128.

SAGHIR, M., and ROBINS, E. 1973. *Male and Female Homosexuality*. Baltimore: Williams & Wilkins.

STOLLER, R. 1968. *Sex and Gender: On the Development of Masculinity and Femininity*. New York: Science House.

YALOM, I., GREEN, R., and FISK, N. 1973. Prenatal exposure to female hormones: Effect on psychosexual development in boys. *Arch. Gen. Psychiatry*, 28:554-561.

YOUNG, W., GOY, R., and PHOENIX, C. 1964. Hormones and sexual behavior. *Science*, 143:212-218.

Part VI
SPECIAL RESEARCH PROBLEMS

15

Responses of the Preschool Child to Divorce: Those Who Cope

JUDITH S. WALLERSTEIN, M.S.W.

In previous papers (Wallerstein and Kelly, 1974, 1975, 1976; Kelly and Wallerstein, 1976) we have reported the research design and the preliminary findings from an ongoing longitudinal study of the effects of parental divorce on 131 children and adolescents drawn from a nonclinic population in a suburban community in northern California. The forum for the first presentation of our data was an international conference in 1974, convened to consider children at risk.* Accordingly, we chose to examine first the children who seemed in significantly worsened psychological condition at the time of the first follow-up, one year after our initial assessment (Wallerstein and Kelly, 1975). In this paper I will discuss that cohort of preschool children who were judged, a year later, to be maintaining their previous good developmental pace, or appeared well on their way to recovery from an acute depressive or regressive reaction to the stresses of the family rupture and to the resumption of their developmental

This research has been supported since 1971 by the Zellerbach Family Fund, San Francisco. The project staff consisted of Mrs. Wallerstein, principal investigator; Joan B. Kelly, Ph.D., co-principal investigator; Angela Homme, Ph.D.; Doris Juvinall Schwarz, M.S.W.; Susannah Roy, M.S.W.; Janet West, M.S.W. A full report of the project will appear in the book, *Children of Separation and Divorce* by Judith S. Wallerstein and Joan B. Kelly, to be published by Basic Books, Inc., New York.

* Congress of the International Association for Child Psychiatry and Allied Professions, Philadelphia, Pa., July, 1974, "The child in his family: Children at psychiatric risk."

agendas or who were, in some instances, showing a developmental spurt and quickening.

Of the entire sample, a total of 34 children, 18 boys and 16 girls, were between the ages of two-and-a-half years and five years, 11 months. All of these children, as we have already described (Wallerstein and Kelly, 1975), suffered intensely from fear, bewilderment, worry, and profound sorrow at the disruption of their families. Fifteen of the 33 whom we reached at the first follow-up (45 percent) seemed significantly worse when reassessed a year later. These comprised five out of 17 of the boys (29 percent) and a dismaying 10 out of 16 of the girls (63 percent). In addition, four children (12 percent) were placed in an intermediate category and were considered to be adequately holding at their previous, somewhat precarious, psychological state. This report concerns the remaining 14 of the 33 (42 percent), nine boys and five girls, who appeared to have coped successfully with the stresses of the family rupture and competently negotiated the many obstacles of the first-year adjustment within the postseparation family—in brief, those children whose distress did not eventuate in developmental interference which could be discerned at that time.

Begun in 1971, the Children of Divorce Project has, as its overarching goals, the systematic exploration of the differential responses of children at various ages to divorce-related family change, as well as to those changes that occur consequent to the divorce within the parent-child relationship. This inquiry represents a first in-depth look at children of divorce drawn from a normal, in the sense of nonclinical, child population. Before the family disruption, all of these children had been considered by their parents and teachers to have reached appropriate developmental milestones. The children and their families were seen individually through the lens of clinical interviews averaging 14.2 interviews per family, extending over a six-week span, set within the context of a preventively oriented planning service which was established by the Project at the county community mental health center. Families were referred by attorneys, schools, physicians, and other community agencies within no more than a year after the parental separation and preferably as close as possible to that separation. Initial data obtained in these four to six interviews with each family member over a six-week period were supplemented by independent information obtained from the children's schools. All family members were interviewed again individually by the same member of the interdisciplinary clinical team, within about a year following this initial extended contact. For most of the families, the follow-up occurred, therefore, at about 18 months after the parental separation.

In consideration of the extraordinary high return of the families for follow-up (58 of the original 60 families) and the finding of such high incidence of continuing or increased distress among the children, we decided to follow the original group further, and in 1976 completed another round of examination of the same youngsters, now four to five years older. Some of the data from the second follow-up are included in this paper.

In earlier reports we stated that decline among the preschool children was not associated with the degree of escalating turmoil before or surrounding the divorce decision, or with the subsequent full-time employment of the custodial parent (most often the mother), if good caretaking arrangements were available to the child. Rather, it appeared that decline in the preschool children seemed linked to the psychological and social ambience of the entire postseparation year, and more specifically to fragility, serious instability, frenetic activity, or depression in the custodial parent, or to unremitting anger between the divorcing spouses which encompassed the child— in brief, with seriously diminished parenting (sometimes unavoidably so). Decline appeared linked, as well, to the intolerable pain of rejection or desertion by the departing parent. In addition, we found that children age three to five, especially little girls, were particularly vulnerable to the effects of the family disruption which appeared to pose a grave threat to their self-esteem, as well as to school adjustment and early learning.

The task of identifying and understanding the children who coped successfully has been even more difficult in that it brings together a host of major unresolved theoretical issues in our field. Existing knowledge of pathology and breakdown is considerably greater than the understanding of stress resistance and the recovery process. As White and his co-workers stated in 1973, "Nowhere in the literature could we find a detailed description of a healthy, well-developed six-year-old human" (White et al., 1973).

Further, it is well known that some loss of function occurs in all children in the face of threatening experience. The operation of stress as a challenge evoking greater efforts at mastery is little understood. And beyond these considerations, individual variations in coping style, idiosyncratic patterns of recovery, and different developmental time tables that are affected by biological, psychological, and social parameters interacting complexly make it difficult to delineate linkages and causal sequences.

Lois Murphy (1976) recently distinguished two major strands of the coping process: by coping I she means the capacity to cope with opportunities, challenges, frustrations, and threats in the environment; this she differentiates from coping II which she defines as the capacity to maintain internal integration in the face of stress. Although it overlaps in some significant regards, the distinction has particular relevance to children of divorce because of the wide range and subtlety of the possible psychological sequelae to the family disruption. Obviously, coping which is immediately or soon evident in successes in school, in relationships with peers and adults, and in the relative absence or brief duration of serious psychological and physical symptoms is easier to observe, to compare, and even to measure. The capacity to maintain inner integrations is stickier, in that it speaks to issues of capacity to overcome severe disappointment and rejection and a host of anxieties without the impairment of the child's potential for spontaneity, loving, appropriate anger, and compassion in his continuing emotional and moral growth. Many of these observations can be made only within the context of a close, intimate relationship that has developed over time.

For our judgment of competent outcome, we have, therefore, attempted a combination of methodological approaches. We have used clinically derived criteria, employing as a measure the comparative judgment of the same examiner, assessing each child against the baseline of how he or she appeared to the same therapist a year later in the context of the clinical relationship. In addition, all of the children we considered improved met accepted developmental norms which reflect age-appropriate and socially expected educational, intellectual, and social achievements.*

Important in this context is our insistence on the developmental perspective as the touchstone of our assessment of the kinds of enduring resolutions achieved by these children of divorce. In this regard, any single cross-sectional vantage point can, by itself, be deceptive for assesment purposes—for example, the lesser visibility of the feeling life, especially the more tender feelings of the child that is such a usual characteristic of latency as a developmental phase. And even more crucial as a reason for long-range follow-up and perspective is our growing awareness that long-range continuities in development are less established than we once thought, and that so many of the circumstances that might elicit creative or deleterious consequences of the childhood trauma, like the challenge and the stress of being oneself a marital partner and a parent, lie in the distant future for these young subjects and are plainly not predictable in any way from our knowledge at this time. Given these considerations, our research strategy has been that of stepwise assessment of the progression through and the mastery within each successive developmental phase, in each instance as measured against the normative standards we have for it.

My goal in this paper is to delineate some of the salient differences that obtained in the family relationships of the children who improved, as against those whose condition worsened. I shall attempt, as well, to note the supports which the improved children had available to them, or which they themselves constructed in their seemingly successful efforts to maintain their developmental course. Finally, the initial responses of both groups will be compared; some of the psychological attributes and psychic mechanisms that characterize these improved children's efforts to cope will be noted, together

---

* The children judged to be competent also met most of the criteria described by Garmezy and Nuechterlein (1972) in their detailed summary of the literature, both published and unpublished, on competent economically disadvantaged children.

with the possible psychological cost to the child of successful adaptation to family rupture.

THE YOUNGEST PRESCHOOL GROUP

The youngest children in our preschool group, who were between two years, six months and three years, three months when first seen in our project, form a small cluster of nine, four boys and five girls. All of these children initially responded to the family disruption with a wide range of behaviors, including acute regression, heightened aggression and irritability, fearfulness, separation anxiety, bewilderment, acute sadness, and tears. Although the extent and duration of each child's distress and symptoms varied, regressive behavior occurred in all the children with no sex differences noted. Similarity between the responses of these children and those severe responses described by Anna Freud and Burlingham (1943), Bowlby, Robertson, and Rosenbluth (1952), and others following separation of young children from their primary caretakers was observed, although in our sample all but one child remained with the mother in the family home.

The four of these nine children who seemed in reasonably good psychological condition a year after this initial contact (three of five girls and one of four boys) did *not* appear different in their initial reactions from the children whose progress was considered poor. Indeed, for two of the children who were later considered to be doing well, the initial reaction was especially severe because separation of the parents resulted in the loss for them of their primary caretaker, the father for one little girl and the mother for one little boy in this subgroup. The initial response to separation was seen, therefore, to have little predictive or prognostic usefulness at this young age.

All four of the improved children in this youngest preschool group experienced a diminution of turmoil in the parental struggles and increased order in their homes during the intervening year. This is in accord with the findings of Hetherington, Cox, and Cox (1975) that the household disorder usually peaks at about one year postseparation. By contrast, the intensity and sense of ongoing conflict and/or depression were relatively unchanged or even heightened in the home of the three children who appeared worse at follow-up. Although still unsettled in their various new roles, three mothers of the improved children had nevertheless begun to make progress in jobs, in return to school, and in finding new and more gratifying social and sexual relationships. The one custodial father, although still in distress, had gradually during the year come to terms with the finality of the divorce he had not wanted. These four custodial parents had established adequate caretaking arrangements for the children, routines had become reestablished, and life had become a reasonably predictable experience. Visits with the noncustodial father were regular and emotionally supportive for two of the children. Although two others continued to feel disappointed in the relative disinterest of the visiting parent and the infrequency of the visits, there was no outright rejection or desertion.

All of these custodial parents had, in response to our brief six-week intervention, been able to modify their behaviors with their children in ways that would assure the child of the parent's continued caretaking and concern. Our data indicate that the parents of the children who improved were those who were able to make good use of our counseling and, by the same token were, perhaps, parents who brought psychological intactness and sensitivity to their parenting role, despite their sometimes distraught behavior at that time. Contrariwise, the parents of the children who got worse had difficulty in using advice constructively. For example, one mother of a severely depressed child rejected our suggestion that the father's departure be discussed with the boy, insisting that he was too young to understand.

Perhaps the central point of difference of the children's experience in these two groups was the fact that the parents of the children who improved did not place the child centrally in the continuing parental struggles. The parents of the improved children were able to maintain a relative separation between their needs and ego boundaries and the needs and ego boundaries of the children. Two parents of the children who did poorly in this group brought their children into the orbit of their anger and depression and maintained the young child as their constant and often only companion. A third mother seemed, in her restless agitation, almost oblivious to the needs of her children and was angrily arranging a move to a distant city, with no plans for continued contact with the children's father who had been visiting regularly.

The stability of the environment of these four improved children can at best be considered marginal, and their improvement, therefore, may reflect as well the stress resistance and coping capacities of the children themselves. As judged at the one-year follow-up, their environment still held many risks. Thus, one child had been left by his mother and was being cared for by his devoted but hard-working father, at great psychic cost to the father; three mothers were working full-time for long hours, with limited skills and poor pay. Two of the improved children were repeatedly hurt and disappointed in their relationship with the visiting father.

The complexity of the task, the successful struggle of the child, as well as the possible psychic cost to the child, are illustrated by Karen who was two-and-a-half years old at the initial contact. After her parents separated, Karen regressed in her toilet training, exhibited frequent temper tantrums, refused to eat her breakfast, exhibited irritability, whining, demanding, clinging behavior, and a profound sadness accompanied by silent crying when alone in her room. To the bewilderment of her mother, she became suddenly preoccupied with staking out claims throughout her world, asserting crossly "This is mine. That is mine." Karen and her hard-pressed mother were locked into an escalating cycle of frustration and mutual irritation which peaked daily when the mother returned from work. Her father, who had been a major parenting figure, visited irregularly.

A year later, Karen at age three-and-a-half appeared bright, lively, outgoing, and fairly sunny. Still in a somewhat unstable living arrangement, she was dividing her week among the separate homes of her two parents and her baby-sitter, spending several days each week with her mother who worked full time, several with her father and his steady girlfriend, and all day long some days in the home of her baby-sitter. She seemed able to make these complex transitions without visible strain and with a clear sense of reality that astonished us in such a young child. She volunteered cheerily, referring to her father's female friend, "I have two mommies and one daddy." In an extraordinary summary of her situation and functioning, she balanced a little toy chair perilously on the gabled roof of the dollhouse, noting "It's safe. It won't fall." The child's relationship with both parents was improved at one year. The father had resumed an important role in her care, and the mother, with considerable advice from us which she had been able to use well, had deescalated her own activities and organized her life with the child. The mother also was beginning to feel both relief and some happiness in her work and her social life, although she was still under considerable pressure.

Seen almost three years later, Karen appeared to be a bright, assertive, no-nonsense, sturdy six-year-old. She aggressively explored the consulting room in its entirety, playing every game in the office. To our surprise, she remembered the dollhouse and the toys. More to our surprise, she remembered the house where she had lived before her parents separated, when she was two years and one month old. She recalled their fights at that time. She said, matter-of-factly and without discernible sadness, that her parents still fight: "I'm used to it. They just don't like each other at all. They even fight over what's good for me. I'm used to that, too." She added, with some disdain, "They fight over little things." When asked what she does when they fight, she retorted, "What do you think I do? I leave the room, of course." The only clue she gave to continued underlying upset was her response when asked for advice regarding what to tell a six-year-old whose parents were undergoing divorce. She hesitated considerably and then offered, "I'd tell her a joke, or make her laugh. I don't like to see children unhappy. It makes me nervous." At school, Karen was reported to be an excellent student but given to tense, shrill verbal outbursts and having some difficulty in making and holding friends. The teacher found that she could calm the child best by placing her on her lap and did so on occasion. The school was also aware that the child spent a lot of time after school without adequate supervision, and that she sometimes came to school without lunch, at which time the teachers scurried about to provide for her. Sometimes the child would suddenly make remarks to the teacher: "My mother bought me 15 dresses yesterday." Or, "My mother gave me lots of money yesterday. Just lots and lots." The teacher had been moved to considerable caring and compassion by what she sensed as Karen's loneliness. Some mothers in the neighborhood will not permit their children to play with Karen because, in their view, she has so little supervision.

This case highlights several conceptual issues in this subsample of the children who improved. Karen has, in accord with the criteria of White et al. (1973) which emerged in their observation of competent preschool children, been able to get and maintain adult attention, to use adults as resources, to learn well, to show pride in her achievement, and to express a desire and interest in growing up. Or, in terms of Murphy's (1976) conception of coping I, Karen has demonstrable competence in her capacity to deal successfully with her environment, in response to the perceived threat. Specifically, Karen makes good use of her intelligence, perceptiveness, clarity, excellent memory, aggressiveness, courage, and flexibility, and of her capacity to reach out and maintain emotional contact with people. Yet, she has been and remains lonely and at times intensely unhappy. Much of her neediness, her unfulfilled longing to be cared for, her desperate concern with what belongs reliably and predictably to her, is in the process of being covered up, denied, and transmuted into a bratty, sometimes hard, sometimes jaunty early independence, reflected in her manner and in her precocious, almost adolescent, jaundiced view of her parents. Her interviewer remarked wryly, "This is no child to entrust with family secrets at a party." Karen's need to avoid and deny emerges most clearly in her suggestion that the unhappy child whose parents are divorcing should be told a joke, as well as in her sudden assertions to the teacher of her mother's extraordinary indulgence and bounty. We may ask, what is this youngster's capacity to be responsive to her own feelings, to her needs for comforting, to many needs that remain unmet? To what extent, also, is it possible for Karen and other children like Karen to receive from other adults, namely from teachers and other people in their environment, the affectionate care and consistent concern that Karen feels are lacking in significant ways at home, despite the efforts of both her parents and their genuine, albeit conflicted, concern and affection?

Finally, we must ask, at what point in her development is it appropriate to observe and assess outcome? For example, the degree to which Karen's defensiveness is related to her entry into latency and her consequent need to resist regressive pulls and reject intense feelings may only become evident from the hindsight of observation in later life stages.

Karen's overall psychic state at this time can best be summarized by her parting story at our last interview. She drew a building on the blackboard and told the following story: "It's a hospital. A little boy just came home from the hospital. He was hit by a car, but now he's OK." And she sailed out.

If we look at the other improved children in this youngest subgroup, at least three are bright and perceptive and well able to make use of language to communicate with their parents and with us. "Daddy, let's have another talk," Jimmy said, as he started to cry on the way home from their visit with his mother. These children showed a good sense of reality discrimination and seemed able at an early age to separate fantasy and reality. They did not seem to take blame for the divorce in their family. We were somewhat surprised at their responsiveness and pleasure in their contacts with us, some of which must also have been evident in their relationships with their teachers and baby-sitters and may well have resulted in the development of their own support system. Only a few weeks after his mother had suddenly left the family, Jimmy, with sweetness and not a little flirtatiousness, threw his arms around the interviewer and surprised her with a kiss as he left his second hour. All of these children struggled hard to understand and explain the family disruption and to deal with the loss. They used projection: "My sister is a crybaby. *She* cries for my daddy." They used denial through fantasy: "My daddy sleeps in my bed every night." But when pushed, the child admitted sadly, "I don't really see him enough." They reversed the loss and transformed it into a gain: "I have two families

now. I have two mommies and one daddy." And they held stead-
fastly and loyally to their relationship with their mothers and fathers.
Karen rejected her mother's boyfriend's overtures crossly: "You are
not my daddy!" Among the responses we saw at the end of the first
year in many of the improved children were stoical acceptance, courage, early independence, sometimes brattiness, and early capacity to
modulate needs and feelings in relation to others, and a capacity to
bear loneliness and psychic hurt without enduring regression.

THE MIDDLE PRESCHOOL GROUP

The middle preschool group consisted of 11 children, five boys
and six girls, age three years, nine months to four years, 10 months
at the time of the first assessment. Although the turmoil around these
children was moderate and no custody battles were threatened, the
incidence of poor outcome in this group was dismayingly high. Seven
of the ten children whom we reached at follow-up, two boys and
five girls, were worse than when first seen. Three children appeared
better: two boys and one girl. And of these, one boy who had initially
been considered by us in serious psychological difficulty, had been
referred at the assessment time for psychotherapy. Accurately, therefore, only two children of 11, one boy and one girl, in this middle
preschool group can be considered within a category of relative stress
resistance.

The two children shared at the outset the worries, fears, and pre-
occupations of their peers who became worse. Like all the children
in this group, they, too, were initially painfully bewildered by the
family disruption, and frightened at what they considered to be their
own replaceability and the possible loss of the remaining custodial
parent. Unlike the other children in this group, these two children
who improved seemed less blaming of themselves for the family disruption and the father's departure.

Frank was one of the children who improved. First seen at age
four years-three months, Frank had been his mother's favorite child,
and his self-esteem, although shaken, was still high. At the time that
we saw him, he was frightened. He was fearful of losing both parents

and had become clinging, tearful, petulant, and sulky at home. He refused to discuss the family rupture with our interviewer and denied any unhappiness, although he was obviously in considerable psychic pain. He offered, with a conscious effort to save face, "I don't miss my father. I see him all the time. It's just like always." Our gentle efforts to probe led him to question his mother on the way home from the interview. He asked, "Is Daddy going to get another wife? Another dog? Another little boy? Who is to blame?" Although he allowed himself to ask these questions of his mother, at no time with us or with his mother did he express the many acute feelings attached to these questions. Throughout his several hours of contact with us, Frank produced many drawings of animals, of flowers, sometimes a family portrait that included both parents. Otherwise he spent his time straightening up the office, lining up pens, papers, and toys in rows to his liking. We were interested in his nonexpression of fears, angers, or concerns directly, either in conversation, play, or art, and his use of the office as a microcosm in which he could reestablish the order, continuity, familiarity, and control that were absent in his world at that time. We were also interested that he complained when his sessions ended.

By the first follow-up, Frank had reorganized. He appeared charming, confident, calm, serious, and poised. He seemed to have made an early entry into latency, was proficient in sports and considered an excellent student. He was intensely competitive in school and with his peers.

Frank was age eight and in third grade when he was seen again in the second follow-up. He had sustained severe stresses in his life in the intervening years, including one parent's major operation. He had begun to show some strain, which was reflected in complaints of fatigue, difficulty in concentrating at school, and preoccupation with fantasy superheroes. Yet, in all, he was still doing exceedingly well. He had entered a new class that year, in a new school, with very aggressive boys who banded together to exclude him. Frank had learned judo, and by the end of the year had established himself by "socking a kid in the mouth." His intense competitiveness with peers continued in school and on the playground. He was described as having good relationships with parents and teachers. The interviewer commented, "Frank struck me as a fine boy with a great deal of intelligence, sensitivity, and good looks. Yet, I missed a sense of humor and the playlike features that one finds in many eight-year-olds whom I see. His pleasures seem tied to competition—hard competition— and winning." When asked for advice for a child whose parents were divorcing, Frank said seriously and stoically, "I'd tell the kid to live with it (the divorce)—to try not to worry. It will turn out OK." For the parents, he advised, "Take care of him. Have fun for him. Have some treats for him, too." Frank also raises issues similar to those represented in Karen, namely, the question of the extent to which his capacity for pleasure and play may have been sapped by his extraordinary and successful response to the many severe stresses of these past few years. His intense competitiveness and drive to win may have served him in good stead in maintaining his developmental course. They may propel him to very high achievements but may also have a psychological toll, whose full effects on his emotional life and capacity for contentment may not yet be evident.

Although we shall not attempt to generalize about this group from these two children, Frank also illustrates one of the important findings with these children, namely, that there is little evidence in our study that preschool children who are able to articulate their feelings necessarily do better than those who deny, avoid, or otherwise shy away from such expression. It is difficult to assess how much of any child's behavior reflects restraint, reserve, conscious avoidance, and/ or denial, or an admixture of these. Nevertheless, the fact remains that several of the preschool children who improved were not able or willing, in their contacts with us, to express in play or conversation or drawing the feelings that could be inferred from their tenseness, restlessness, and symptomatic behaviors. Our evidence is that they did not talk to other adults, either, at this time.

These improved or stress-resistant children, by and large, did have, in our experience, a remarkably clear and differentiated perception of happenings in their particular world and of many of the details and implications of the family rupture. This clarity was often not found in their peers who did poorly, in whom we more often found a denial of the events, a clinging to fantasy remarriage or reconciliation, and a lack of clarity in separating wishes from reality. It seems important, in this regard, to distinguish denial of the reality from denial of painful feelings or fears. It is possible that the improved children are those who are able to be clear about the reality but are able, often, to avoid, deny, conceal, or otherwise dose or titrate their painful feelings until they feel able to deal with these in their own good time. These observations have obvious implications for clinical assessment as well as for program. It is important to intervention theory that such avoidance or denial of feelings at the initial contact, namely at the time when the stress is at its height, is not predictive either of the adjustment at a later date, or of the later capacity to deal wih these feelings successfully.

THE OLDEST PRESCHOOL GROUP

The oldest group of preschool children included 14, nine boys and five girls, who were between the ages of five years and five years-11 months at the initial assessment. At the time of the parental separation, many of these children experienced heightened anxiety and aggression, which became manifest in their restlessness, whininess, moodiness, general irritability, and symptomatic behaviors that included phobias, sleep disturbances, compulsive eating, aggressive outbursts, and a driven search for physical contact and attention from adults. These initial responses to the family rupture seemed more diverse, from the outset, when compared with those of the younger children.

In addition, one of the distinguishing attributes of this older preschool group was the greater consistency between their predominant psychological stance at first observation and the characteristic patterning of defensive and coping mechanisms evident at the year's end. The children who were worse at follow-up were, with one exception, very troubled at the initial counseling. Similarly, all but one child in this age group were improved or in relatively good shape at the initial counseling. Therefore, these initial clinical findings may have somewhat greater predictive value and can, perhaps, be used somewhat more reliably for early intervention and referral than those of the two younger preschool groups.

Several of the oldest children seemed, from the start, capable of maintaining some degree of psychological distance or perspective vis à vis the parental conflict. One boy expressed what seemed to be genuine relief at being separated from his father. Several others, despite their anxiety, sadness, and anger, appeared able to continue their lives in school, play, and with peers without significant impediment. At follow-up, these children were members of the group that was doing well. In all, seven of the 14 children in this older preschool group (50 percent), six boys and one girl, may be considered to come within a subgroup of stress-resistant children who had indeed been able to experience the family separation and the ensuing year of disequilibrium without evident long-term detriment to their psychological development. The vulnerable children included four girls and one boy who appeared significantly worse at the first follow-up, and two additional children, both boys, who continued to appear as vulnerable at follow-up as they had at the earlier examination, although they had not lost ground.

Much like that of the younger improved children, the mother-child relationship of these improved youngsters seemed to have improved by follow-up. The intense turmoil and parental fighting present in five of the seven children's families at the time of the initial evaluation had diminished. And in all except one of the families, the mother was feeling better than at the time of the initial examination.

Several of these mothers had special relationships with the boys who improved. Of the six boys in the improved group of older preschool boys, three were the only boys in a sibship of three and enjoyed a preferred relationship with their mothers, especially when compared with their older sisters, whose relationship with their mothers was burdened by overt conflict and anger. The pattern of preferential treatment of the boy was particularly evident in the two families in which the one boy was also the youngest child. The one girl in this group of children who improved was also the youngest child and had been, from the start, closely identified with her mother. Her older brother was encountering considerable difficulty in his adjustment in the family.

Yet, by and large, it should be said that most of the six mothers of the improved children were undergoing considerable stress in the year following the parental separation. Only one mother was, in fact, competent and intact in her functioning at follow-up. Three mothers had a history of serious somatic illness complicated by psychological components and sequelae. Two mothers among the three had sought the divorce after painfully extricating themselves from a humiliating marriage in which they had suffered physical and psychic abuse over many years. A fifth woman was suffering from chronic depression. At least two of these families were in serious economic straits; three mothers had begun to work for the first time after the parental separation; all but two were worried about finances. Yet, with one exception, none of these women burdened their children's visitation with their fathers, nor were the children subjected to criticism or rejection if they expressed interest or eagerne s in seeing their fathers. In brief, these children were not made to feel central in the continuing parental struggles, despite resentments that continued to smolder in four of the six families.

Of the six oldest preschool boys who improved or held onto previous good adjustment, two openly regarded the diminished contact with the father as an opportunity to establish a not unwelcome distance. David, age five, the youngest of four children, had been the object of his father's most significant attachment during the marriage, as well as the target of his frequent, bitterly sarcastic, critical outbursts. His mother attributed the deterioration of the marriage in part to parental rivalry over the child's affection. David appeared, in his initial contact with us, as a whiny, immature, unhappy little boy who was anxiety-ridden at school and on the playground and stridently tyrannical at home. After the parental separation, the father began to visit weekly, but his visits included all of the siblings together, and the relationship with David became, as a result, less intense, less all-encompassing, and less geared to serving the father's changing moods and pressing needs. David expressed satisfaction with this new arrangement. At the end of the first year, the boy appeared to have made almost two years of growth; he was significantly freer to use aggression in his relationship with his peers, considerably less fearful, and surging ahead in academic and social learning. At the four-year mark, the report we have indicates that the boy, now age nine, is still doing splendidly and is a source of pride to his mother and his teachers. Before the second follow-up, the family had been living for several years at a considerable distance from the father. It may well be that circumscribing the pathological relationship with the father has promoted this youngster's development.

If one looks at the quality of relationship between these fathers and the improved subgroup of oldest preschool boys, it seems that four among six had fathers whose relationships with these children were profoundly disturbed. The attenuation of these relationships, however painful to the children, may have nevertheless set the children free from bonds that were impeding their developmnt. All but one of the children in this subgroup saw their fathers four times a month during the first year. None of these fathers deserted or overtly rejected their children. One father moved to a distant city and saw his son on holidays and weekends. The father's relationship with the one little girl in this improved group was closer and warmer at follow-up than at the time of the separation, when he refused to visit for several months because of his pain and jealousy.

Of the three mothers who had remarried at the time of the first follow-up, two of the children had important and loving relationships with their stepfathers. For example, Frances, whose mother remarried shortly after the divorce, acquired a new stepfather and several older brothers at the same time. Frances occupied a special place in this household as the only girl and the youngest child. This role seemed to enhance her feminine identification as well as her closeness to her mother. The child's unusual prettiness, charm, and warmth were significant factors in evoking the gratifications she received.

At least three of the children in this oldest preschool group seemed to have been protected from the pressure of parental needs and from exposure to parental violence and seduction by the presence of another sibling who more directly sustained the pressures of the parental needs and conflicts. It is of interest that of two brothers in one family in this oldest preschool group, the older boy showed signs of considerable psychological deterioration at the end of the first year, whereas the younger one seemed to have negotiated the year's hurdles with more success. Of seven improved children in this older preschool group, six had older siblings of whom three were more troubled youngsters, and two additional older siblings were locked in angry conflicts with the parents which seemed to have been precipitated or exacerbated by the family separation. (Of the two children who improved in the middle preschool group, both children had older siblings, one of whom was in considerable psychological trouble, and the other suffered with a chronic physical disability.)

Academically and socially, the seven improved children in this older preschool group were doing well at follow-up. One child had a minor speech problem for which he was in therapy, and another seemed to have some minor reading difficulty. Three of the children about whom there had been mixed reports at the time of the initial evaluation were now considered excellent students. Larry, for example, whose teacher had reported mood swings, day-dreaming, and reading difficulties at the time of the first assessment, was considered a model student at follow-up. By and large, these children related well to peers and to their teachers. These reports stand sharply in contrast with the findings regarding the children in this age group who deteriorated, where we were particularly concerned with the number of serious learning difficulties and disturbed relationships with peers.

It also seems clear that these children were using their relationships with teachers and other students to provide themselves with needed supports and, in effect, to construct their own support systems. This emerged in part from the pleasure and warmth with which many of their teachers discussed these youngsters. Furthermore, the reports on these children who were doing well at school were sometimes at minor variance with their behavior at home, suggesting that these children were able to shift their behavior in response to the demands and gratifications of the setting. Our finding regarding the significance of the school in providing support for these children has important implications for the school and for the teacher.

It seems that the school and the classroom often provide the only continuity available to the child at the time of the divorce.

In noting other support systems available, it should be mentioned that a somewhat higher percentage of these children than the children who did poorly had grandparents who were concerned with their welfare and were helpful to the children directly or to the custodial parent. Two of the extended families lived close by, and the children visited them frequently. Others provided vacation homes and financial help.

An accelerated push toward increased maturity seems to characterize the older preschool children who improved. In a sense, their turning away from the stresses of the family disruption, and their wish to escape the conflicts between their parents, moved them more quickly into the next developmental stage, whose hallmarks are increased independence from the family, diminution in the intensity of parent-child relationships, and movement outward toward school and playground with new adult models and new peers. It may be that the departure of the oedipal father accelerated this outward movement in these children, in part as a result of their need to avoid the danger of a regressive pull to the relationship with a reactivated pre-oedipal mother, as well as the danger of being left alone with a powerful oedipal mother who had, in several of these children's fantasies, banished the father and won the family turf. It should be noted that this increased independence represents, as well, an adaptive response to diminished caretaking. Hetherington, Cox, and Cox (1975) reported that young children of recently separated parents are more likely than children of married parents to get pick-up meals, to eat irregularly, to eat separately from the custodial parent, and to put themselves to bed.

Each of these children seemed able to make his way into the new early-latency territory, to perform at least adequately in various new roles, and to become the kind of child who engenders positive responses from the new adults, in effect to be bright, responsive, highly motivated, and capable of mastering the rules and meeting the requirements of her or his peer society. Moreover, these same children were able to adapt to new stepparents without overwhelming conflict and without sacrificing their attachment to the noncustodial visiting parent. Solnit (1970) has suggested that released aggression may be a significant component in the so-little understood process of recovery. And it may be that these improved children have been able to harness the rising aggression, which we observe in so many children in response to family disruption, to advance their entry into the next developmental phase. If so, their use of newly available aggressive energies, combined with the self-propelled move outward away from the family conflict, would shed some light on what has been observed as a developmental spurt that can occur in response to stress.

It is, of course, not possible at the present time to know whether these adaptive behaviors are the consequence of stress resistance or represent its component parts. Viewed at close range, these children showed the capacity for perception with regard to their families and an ability to accept the family rupture as a reality with a minimum of subterfuge and self-blame. How much of this reflected a conscious, studied scanning of the family landscape is hard to judge. We were often impressed with the acute social sensitivity of these children. Tom drew himself with large eyes and enormous ears, reflecting perhaps both the intensity and the strain of needing constantly to assess the world around him. The children seemed able, despite their own pain, clearly to distinguish their wishes for reconciliation from the reality they perceived. John told us how much he missed his father and how much he wished to live with him. He added, with great sadness, "But, he does not want to live with us any more." The children worked hard at explaining the separation, even when it made no sense to them at all. Frances insisted that her parents divorced because of fights about "mail and taxes." The children made judgments about right and wrong. Tom, who was surrounded by adult violence which included gun possession and threats of killing, told us that it was wrong to give vent to anger. Several children showed a capacity for planful, independent, multistep activities. At follow-up, Frances told us that her remarried mother was working very hard with her newly acquired large family. Therefore she, Frances, had decided to dress herself and do much for her own care, to help her mother. Her perceptions were, like those of her peers, realistic, pragmatic, and detailed.

Of the entire group of 14 improved children at the one-year point, we were able to reach 13 at the four-year mark. For these, our very preliminary analysis reveals that a goodly number of family changes have occurred in their young lives, including several remarriages, a second divorce for one, a pending divorce for another parent, and a partial reconciliation. Only three of the 13 children were found to be in overt distress. The remainder, who were examined by the original clinician, were considered to be still within appropriate developmental norms and doing adequately or well in their psychological and social functioning. All three of the children who had deteriorated in this interval seem profoundly affected by what they felt to be their fathers' disinterest or rejection.

SUMMARY

Of 34 preschool children seen shortly after the parental separation, a total of 14, or 42 percent, seemed one year later to have weathered the initial postseparation period and to have resumed the developmental progress which had been briefly interrupted in most instances. The factors that differentiated the environment of these improved children from that of their peers who fared less well seemed related centrally to the reestablishing of caretaking, reasonable routines, and adequate parenting by the custodial parent. Additional factors that emerged as important in the environment of these improved children included the capacity of the divorcing parents to keep continuing angers and conflicts separate from their relationship with the children; the availability of a good school system and teachers with time and sensitivity to offer individual support and encouragement to the child; appropriate distancing from a pathological parent-child relationship, where this preceded the divorce; and the absence of overt rejection or desertion by either parent. Siblings seemed, as well, to offer a buffering support to younger children, sometimes at the price of their own increased conflict with a distressed parent. Relationships with a stepparent, particularly the marriage partner of the custodial parent, seemed also to have growth-promoting and comforting potential for some children.

The initial responses of the younger preschool children who improved at one year were indistinguishable at that time from those whose psychological and social functioning later declined. By kindergarten age, differences could more often be distinguished at the outset, with the children who declined during the first few months after the separation showing more troubled behavior a year later.

The children who seemed to cope successfully with the stress of the family disruption were intelligent, perceptive, and courageous, and they had the capacity to make do with less time and less caretaking and to become increasingly independent, as well as to develop their own supports outside of the immediate family. They were propelled by this adaptation along the developmental ladder toward greater independence and earlier entry into the next developmental stage. Some seemed able to make this complex adaptation without openly expressing their intense feelings and fears, as long as they were able, cognitively, to face the reality of the divorce and to be assured by trusted parents of continued love and care.

Our findings are that the children who were improved at about 18 months after the parental separation had, by and large, fought a successful battle to overcome their initial acute fright, conflict, self-blame, and grief. As part of this adaptive process, which eventuated in their continued development, they were able to circumscribe, to bypass, or to deny their wishes and/or their expectations for the parenting and caretaking that had been their experience before the family rupture. It seems likely that a significant underlay of sadness, neediness, and unfulfilled longing is a significant aspect of their childhood experience during the several years following the parental divorce. This persistent underlying sadness, combined with early self-reliance and early entry into the next developmental stage, seemed to have important implications for character development, including particularly self-concept and relationships with adults and peers. The limitations of our knowledge, the wide range of individual difference, and the particular restrictions that attach to psychological observation during latency preclude long-range predictions. We will, in future publications, report more fully on outcome, as seen at the four-year mark.

REFERENCES

BOWLBY, J., ROBERTSON, J., and ROSENBLUTH, D. 1952. A two-year-old goes to the hospital. *Psychoanal. Study Child,* 7:89-94.

FREUD, A., and BURLINGHAM, D. 1943. *War and Children.* New York: International Universities Press.

GARMEZY, N., and NUECHTERLEIN, K. 1972. Invulnerable children: The fact and fiction of competence and disadvantage. *Am. J. Orthopsychiatry,* 77:328-329.

HETHERINGTON, E. M., COX, M., and COX, R. 1975. Beyond father absence: Conceptualization of the effects of divorce. Presented to the Society for Research in Child Development, Denver.

KELLY, J., and WALLERSTEIN, J. 1976. The effects of parental divorce: Experiences of the child in early latency. *Am. J. Orthopsychiatry,* 46 (1):20-32.

MURPHY, L. 1976. *Vulnerability, Coping, and Growth.* New Haven: Yale University Press.

SOLNIT, A. 1970. A study of object loss in infancy. *Psychoanal. Study Child,* 25:257-272.

WALLERSTEIN, J., and KELLY, J. 1974. The effects of parental divorce: The adolescent experience. In J. Anthony and C. Koupernik (eds.), *The Child in His Family— Children at Psychiatric Risk,* pp. 479-505. New York: Wiley.

WALLERSTEIN, J., and KELLY, J. 1975. The effects of parental divorce: Experiences of the preschool child. *J. Am. Acad. Child Psychiatry,* 14 (4):600-616.

WALLERSTEIN, J., and KELLY, J. 1976. The effects of parental divorce: Experiences of the child in later latency. *Am. J. Orthopsychiatry,* 46 (2):256-269.

WHITE, B. L., and WATTS, J. C. with I. C. BARNETT, B. T. KABAN, J. R. MARMOR, and B. B. SHAPIRO. 1973. *Experience and Environment,* vol. 1, *The Development of the Young Child: Major Influences,* p. 552. Englewood Cliffs, N.J.: Prentice-Hall.

16

Pregnant Adolescents

MICHAEL BAIZERMAN, Ph.D.

Public and professional discussions about pregnant adolescents, married and unmarried, are increasing. Although these discussions are reminiscent of those of the 1960s, there are some differences which include the current emphases on parenting, on birth defects in babies of adolescent mothers, and on service programs.

The emphasis on parenting is found in the title of the major association of service providers—National Alliance Concerned With School-Age Parents (NACSAP)—and in the substance of Sen. Edward Kennedy's bill, The National School-Age Mother and Child Health Act of 1975.

The emphasis on birth defects is found in the work of the March of Dimes which sponsors workshops and conferences and distributes materials on this subject. Special focus is on the adolescent mother because she is at relatively higher risk than other age-cohort mothers to have an infant with one or more birth defects.

Reports of research concerning pregnant adolescents, their male friends, and programs to help them are heard increasingly at the meetings of lay and professional groups like the American Public Health Association and NACSAP. The Kennedy Foundation joined the federal government in sponsoring several meetings where selected researchers discussed their work and suggested prevention and service ideas. Those who have long been concerned about these young women can feel good about the current discussions, for they were a long time in coming. From my reading and participation, I believe that the range of discourse is broad and its quality high.

293

Yet I think that the substance of these discussions and the unstated, unexamined, and unarticulated assumptions upon which some
of the discussions rest are problematic. This assertion is based on my
own work. In this paper my major focus will be on the relation between research and practice. I believe that we must articulate, analyze, and discuss issues of research and practice so that public and
professional discussion will be informed. This could make what is
good even better by making it different.

I have divided this paper into two parts, the first of which focuses
on the relation between research and practice. The issue here is the
limitations of the normative model of relations between practice
and research. The topic of research utilization is approached ob-
liquely, but an alternative model is presented directly.

The second part deals more directly with pregnant youth, and it
is more playful. It presents, and answers briefly, questions that are
rarely found in the published literature on pregnant youth.

The reader may wonder whether the relative absence of material
about pregnant youth in the first part of this paper means that the
ideas presented have no immediate relevance to practitioners and
researchers concerned about these girls. Obviously, I believe that the
issues are directly and immediately relevant to those concerned about
these young women. Indeed, the ideas to be presented began to be
worked out six years ago when I, a professional social worker with
public health training, was working as a researcher on a study of
services to these girls and as an abstractor of published studies about
pregnant youth (Baizerman et al., 1971). With this prelude, let us
walk into the crucial issue—or swamp.

THE RELATIONS BETWEEN COMMON SENSE, PRACTICE, AND RESEARCH QUESTIONS AND ANSWERS

I want to explore the relations between direct practice and sociobehavioral research by focusing on three processes: asking and answering questions and using research in practice. I chose these foci
because it is in these processes that we find cultural and personal
expectations about the possible usefulness of research for practi-

tioners and a way to join the needs, wants, and work of the practitioner and the researcher.

Practitioner Expectations of Research

To begin with a commonsense question: Why do practitioners want empirical sociobehavioral research to be done concerning pregnant adolescents? One reason is the *practitioners' expectation* that something will be learned during such research that could be useful in direct service to pregnant youth (and/or in a variety of other service-related ways).

The practitioner working with pregnant youth who holds such an expectation could go to a seminar on current studies of pregnant adolescents and could read a large number of research reports and articles reporting research with these girls. Will the practitioner find something useful for his or her practice?

The Research Question

One place in which the practitioner can look for something useful in his practice is the research question, the hypothesis of the study. From this the practitioner can learn whether the researcher was trying to answer a question the practitioner believes is important in his own work. This is the part of a study where the "integration" between practice and research is said to occur.

I will suggest, however, that the research question has only surface usefulness for this determination because practitioners and researchers ask different kinds of questions.

Questions from Research, Practice, Theory, and Common Sense

Research reports commonly contain these phrases: The research question is. . . . The practical question here is. . . . The basic theoretical question is. . . . Based on this study, the research question can be answered thusly. . . . Based on these studies, the practice question can be answered (fully or partly or tentatively) in this way. . . .

The daily work of researchers and practitioners is oriented to asking and answering questions. The questions asked derive from other research, from "theory," from the client we are sitting with, from our conceptions of treatment and service, from our conceptions of people and their problems, from everyday life in our nonprofessional worlds, among many, many other sources.

On the surface, it is hard to distinguish commonsense questions from research questions from practice questions from theory questions, except that the words in some refer to "things" and are more abstract that the words in others, and the words in some are more technical than the words in others.

There are profound differences between these types of questions. The differences are found in the different sets of rules used to decide (a) whether a question can be answered, and (b) what constitutes an answer. These sets of rules are different for commonsense questions and commonsense answers, for research questions and answers, for practice questions and answers, and for theoretical questions and answers. A particular question and answer may be acceptable using one set of rules and unacceptable using another set of rules.

For example, it is a commonsensical question to ask: why did Mary become pregnant? It is common sense to answer: Because John didn't use a contraceptive. The same question can be a practice question: why did Mary become pregnant? It is common to hear practice answers such as these: Because (s)he didn't use contraceptives. . . . Because all her friends were getting pregnant. . . . Because she was acting out her mother's conflicts . . . and so on.

But the same question is not a good research question because in most paradigms (Kuhn, 1970) of empirical sociobehavioral research, "why" questions cannot be answered in any acceptable way (McIver, 1964), particularly if the sample is one person.

Another example is found in "how" questions. It is a commonsensical question to ask: How did Mary become pregnant?, to which a commonsense answer is: She became pregnant by having intercourse with John and by not using contraceptives. It is common to hear the same words in a practice question. As a research question and as a "theoretical" question, "how" has both a commonsense answer and the penultimate scientific answer. To be able to say "how" is to be able to use a set of scientific rules to explain how the occurrence came to be; to answer "how" is to have a scientific theory.

The point that questions from practitioners and researchers only *seem* to be the same or similar can be made in another way.

Cross-Cultural Question-Asking

Consider as cultures the commonsense world, the world of practice, and the world of research and theory. These cultures obviously overlap. Consider the limits of cross-cultural question-asking.

It may seem as if a question asked by someone in one culture would have the same meaning to someone in another culture. It does not, necessarily. It may seem as if researchers sometimes ask practitioner questions. They rarely do, because the researcher asks his questions within a cultural and ideational context, which is different, usually, from that of the practitioner. The words may look as if they make sense across cultures, but the meaning of the words is perceived differently by the researcher and the practitioner.

This difference in meaning is seen, in part, in the different thoughts and behaviors of the researcher and of the practitioner which result from asking the question. To put this another way, the researcher and the practitioner understand the question in different ways.

To practitioners, findings are another location in a study to find ideas that could be used in practice. Let us look briefly at answers to questions.

Question-Answering and the Answers to Questions

Obviously there are different ways in which questions are answered. There are commonsense answers, practice answers, and research answers. There are different sets of rules in each culture for what is accepted as an answer and for the "power" of the answer.

As is true for questions, the English words for answers are the same across the three cultures, although the words have somewhat different meanings in each culture. For example, the word "because" is used in each culture; but "because" has different meanings as part of a commonsense answer, a practice answer, and a research answer.

Research "Findings" as a Type of Answer

Answers to questions in one culture look as if they should have the same meaning (s) in other cultures; they rarely do, either symbolically or functionally. The researcher's answers are his "findings."

Research findings are a *constructed reality* which, by convention, is arrived at in certain ways, holds only under certain conditions, and is located in a certain place in the research report.

The practitioner is taught to believe that the researcher's rules, practices, and conventions are the ones which he too must hold. He is taught to hold these as if he were a researcher. To do this is, paradoxically, to delimit the possible meanings and use the answer could have for his practice.

In other words, practitioners have to make practitioner-sense out of research answers. Practitioner-sense is a different order of meaning than researcher-sense; it is neither higher nor lower, better or worse. It is qualitatively different. It is also normatively different in that it follows a different set of rules. As will be suggested, this set of rules is, again paradoxically, rules of doing research rather than rules of using research findings.

I do not want to get into the issues concerning the way researchers often choose their questions or the issues of why researchers do not often ask practitionerlike questions. Rather, I shall suggest briefly an approach to research utilization by practitioners. Three questions serve to summarize the ideas presented and to link these to the proposed model:

1. Are researchers asking and answering commonsense and practice questions in ways that make sense to practitioners?

2. Can researchers ask and answer commonsense and practice questions in ways that make sense to practitioners?

3. Can (or do) practitioners make sense of the answers researchers give to commonsense and practice questions?

Cross-Cultural Utilization of Questions and Answers in Direct Practice

It is common sense to believe that practitioners can use research answers in their everyday practice. The usual phrase for this is the "utilization of research in practice." This belief is part of an ideology about the relation between research and practice; as a cognitive or social process, it is not at all clear how a practitioner uses research in practice.

Texts about research utilization (Tripod, Fellini, and Meyer, 1969) present a model of utilization which is something like this: One reads a reported study and then assesses the quality of the research using normative criteria of "good" research. If the study is found to be "good," then one looks at several locations in the report to find content which could be utilized in a service context. Once found, this content is then "applied" in practice.

This model begins with the research report. I propose an alternate model, one that begins with the practitioner, presenting only the central ideas of this model.

The practitioner is a reader of the "constructed reality" called a research report; he is an analyst of "secondary data." As a worker/reader, the practitioner reads with a perspective that comes, in part, from his worker situation, the people he is working with (or planning for). The worker/reader likely has in mind a question that may be stated this way: Is there something in this study I can use in my work? This and similar questions define the utilization context or utilization situation.

The utilization context is the cognitive context for reading. The context may be "focused" or "unfocused," depending upon whether the worker/reader has in mind a particular or a general-practice situation.

In focused utilization, the worker/reader begins a situation-specific search for items in a study that may be of use to him in a particular practice situation. In unfocused utilization, the reader is scanning, doing reconnaissance for words, ideas, or other items that in general may be of some use in practice at some unspecified time in some unspecified situation.

The worker/reader may choose material from any location within a research report. He is not bound to utilize only the broad research question or hypothesis or the research findings.

Once the worker/reader finds an item he thinks may be of use in practice, he formulates—consciously or not—a utilization hypothesis. This hypothesis is a statement of the worker/reader's judgment that a given item in a study may be of use in a practice situation. This hypothesis is "tested" in practice.

Practice is a research-like process, not a process of applied theory or applied research. The worker proceeds as a worker/researcher doing grounded theory research (Glaser and Strauss, 1967).

In short, it is argued that the normative criteria for assessing the quality of empirical studies may be inappropriate to the process by which practitioners use in their everyday work items from research reports.

In closing this section, I will pose a question about research utilization: Can a worker use in practice a research report published in a 1946 issue of the *American Journal of Orthopsychiatry* about the use of groups in the treatment of juvenile delinquents?

Summary

There are real differences between questions asked and answers given within and between the cultures of commonsense thinking, practice thinking, and research thinking.

These differences in the normative practices of asking and answering questions have important consequences for attempts to work across cultures. This is seen particularly in attempts by practitioners to use research findings in their everyday work.

These issues seem to be among the unstated assumptions that underlie much of the public and professional discussion and exhortation about pregnant adolescents. They are found particularly in the expectation that sociobehavioral research as now carried on will contribute to the solution of the problem and problems of pregnant girls. This neopositivism must be held to less dearly.

SOME FOCUSED QUESTIONS ABOUT PREGNANT ADOLESCENTS

This is the part of the paper in which there are few word games or Talmudic analyses.

I want to raise some questions about pregnant adolescents so as to stimulate, if you will, practice and research.

What is Known About Premature Grandparents and Grandparenting?

The parents of adolescent mothers are grandparents. Very often, these grandparents are between 30 to 45 years old. Given the age-norms associated with our social conceptions of grandparents, these are "premature" grandparents. Little is known about these people and few programs offer services to them.

It would be valuable to study these young grandparents for several reasons. First, we could learn more about the intergenerational family from the points of view of adolescent-pregnancy etiology and child-rearing. Second, we could learn about our conceptions of aging and of grandparenting with an eye to sorting age, physiological change, and sociopsychological status. This is a socially deviant grandparent group.

From a service perspective, it may be that girl-parent relationships are a more effective focus than girl-man relationships if the intent is to enhance the opportunities for healthy development of the youth and the infant.

Such a focus can follow from classical Freudian conceptions of adolescent-pregnancy etiology or from a variety of other conceptions of etiology or service.

Do Girls at the Age of Onset of Menses Understand the Idea of Prevention?

This is a complex question. Five sets of facts and ideas contribute to the question.

First, there are data from large-scale studies that suggest that the chronological age at which menarche occurs has dropped over the last 100 years and is now in the range of 9 to 11 years. Second, there are concepts in the literature about adolescence that suggest that this period of life is characterized in part by a sense that certain things "which could happen to others won't happen to me." Third, there is a set of rules about statistical-probability theory that contributes to a philosophical world view. This view sees the world "probabilistically"—as in the idea that this *may* happen and in the idea that the odds that this will happen are greater than the odds that this will not happen. Fourth, there is a huge literature on adolescent cognitive development. According to Piaget, adolescence is in part that time during which the individual can for the first time do certain mental operations that he could not do before. The fifth set of items is about prevention. In public health, prevention may be primary, secondary, or tertiary. The idea may be divided in other ways: (a) do x to make y happen, (b) don't do x to make y happen, (c) do x to keep y from happening, (d) don't do x to keep y from happening. For *x* one may substitute a variety of health and medical practices, from brushing one's teeth or taking a prescribed or proscribed drug to using a contraceptive. Similarly, one may substitute a variety of outcomes, diseases, or disabilities for *y*.

Now to put these together and to show the source of the question. To rephrase the original question: Do girls before or just after the onset of menses have the cognitive developmental ability to understand the probabilistic nature of primary pregnancy prevention?

Or, phrasing the idea another way: Do nine- to eleven-year-old boys and girls understand that if the odds are ten to one that they will become pregnant if contraceptives are not used (*ceritus parabus*) during sexual intercourse, this does *not* mean that they can have unprotected sexual intercourse nine times without getting pregnant?

The "Why" Question Revisited: Why Don't Some Girls Get Pregnant?

In the first part of this paper I suggested the methodological problems in sociobehavioral research that arise when one uses those approaches to answer a "why" question with a sample of one case. Let's change the "why" question to a "why not" question.

Rather than ask, why did Mary become pregnant?, ask why did Mary not become pregnant? Along with asking, why did these girls become pregnant while those did not?, try asking, why didn't these girls become pregnant while those did?

I suggest that although this simple change in the "why" question may not solve the intricate philosophy of a science question, it might stimulate some different ways of thinking about these girls.

What Is Known About Girls' Phenomenological Conceptions of Health and of Pregnancy?

Very little. It might be of great value to explore this approach to understanding these girls and to offering services to them. Dr. Dale Garrel and associates at the Institute for Humanistic Medicine in San Francisco interviewed young people to learn their understanding of health. They learned it is of a different order than our own; it is on another plane of reality. One youth explained health as playing chess and winning. This is surely not a normative adult professional conception.

The difference should sensitize us to the potential value of this kind of interviewing. The potential of data such as these for treatment and service-planning is obvious, especially if we accept and act on the principle of "starting where the client is." Data such as these tell us where indeed the client really is.

How can we have a program that begins where they are, if we have to write on the grant application to get funds for the program exactly where they are before we see them? I pass! and refer the reader to the "poems" in our recent *Self-Evaluation Handbook for Hotlines and Crisis Centers* (Baizerman, McDonough, and Sherman, 1976).

It is a paradox that can be solved by administrative decision in a framework of "administrative justice."

When Are the Pregnant Girl's Needs Different from Her Wants?

The answer is, when you ask her. Both words, needs and wants, have a long history of use in philosophy, politics, and human services. "Needs" has at least these meanings: *a deficiency,* as when the ideal ratio of physicians to population size is one to 2000 people, but there is only one physician to 10,000 people; *a motive,* as in "he

needed to do that because," or "he did that because his needs were
x and y"; *a moral imperative,* as in "she needs bread" having more
moral weight than "she wants bread"; *a professional (or adult) im-
putation* of cause, as in "I think that the cause of your problem
is ...." "Wants" is a more straightforward political term. It is
a stated desire, one that is legitimate on its face.

The two words, needs and wants, are crucial in discussing pregnant adolescents. We often determine their needs for service and
rarely ask the girl what *she wants.* It is a tough issue, because to
ask and accept in a clinical sense the girl's statement of her wants
often means that her statement will be interpreted with our own
sense of how her want is a need. And around and around.

What Do We Know About Youth's "Folk Wisdom" and Folklore About Pregnancy?

I found very little in the literature about this. I believe that an
anthropological perspective would provide much useful data about
adolescent pregnancy, data necessary for helping girls in clinical
settings and necessary for planning and evaluating service programs.
For example, I have heard girls talk about not going to a dentist
during their pregnancy because of the effects this will have on the
fetus.

Focus would be *not* on the folklore of sexual relations which has
a literature, however rarely used in treatment and service planning,
but on the status of being pregnant. I am searching for data on topics
such as: What does a pregnant girl do and not do, and why? Can a
pregnant girl have sex? Can a young mother have sex after delivery
without worrying about getting pregnant again?

I am suggesting topics that touch on what we call "facts" and what
we call the subjective experience of pregnancy, and suggesting that
we find out whether these have sociocultural sources.

What Do We Know About Teenagers Who Participate in Friend-Assisted Childbirth?

By friend-assisted childbirth I mean programs and techniques such
as those used in Lamaze and the Childbirth Education Association.

I wonder how youth would experience these. The question is intended to stimulate consideration of such a service in programs for youth, and it is also an honest research question. Given the cognitive and psychosocial developmental stages of youth, such a service might provide youth with an opportunity to derive meaning of the pregnancy and birth in unique (i.e., nonadult) ways, which might have important, positive therapeutic consequences.

When Is a Cafeteria a Better Model than a Good Texas Steakhouse?

When one is planning services for pregnant girls.

Don't You Have Any More Questions?

Yes, I do have many more questions that I believe can stimulate research and practice. But I have presented a number of ideas and I am therefore going to stop. Now it's your turn.

REFERENCES

BAIZERMAN, M., McDONOUGH, J. J., and SHERMAN, M. 1976. *Self-Evaluation Handbook for Hotline and Youth Crisis Centers.* St. Paul: Center for Youth Development and Research, University of Minnesota.

BAIZERMAN, M., SHEEHAN, C., ELLISON, D. L., and SCHLESINGER, E. R., 1971. Pregnant adolescents: A review of literature with abstracts, 1960-1970. *Sharing* (Supplement). Washington, D.C.: National Alliance Concerned with School-Age Parents.

GLASER, B., and STRAUSS, A. 1967. *The Discovery of Grounded Theory.* Chicago: Aldine.

KUHN, T. S. 1970. *The Structure of Scientific Revolutions.* Chicago: University of Chicago Press.

McIVER, R. M. 1964. *Social Causation.* New York: Harper & Row.

TRIPODI, T., FELLINI, P., and MEYER, H. J. 1969. *The Assessment of Social Research.* Itasca, Ill.: Peacock.

Index

307